What has been said
about A Caregiver's Guide...

"This Book offers a welcome resource for family caregivers. We congratulate you on producing this excellent document. The caregivers we have worked with often expressed a need for easily understood and readily accessible information to aid them with the new challenges they face. Your guide responds to this need by offering practical, plain-language information about a range of topics—even those issues that are difficult to talk about. More importantly, the information is presented in a sensitive and compassionate manner."

—Marlene MacLellan, Centre of Aging,
Mount St. Vincent University

"This is a wonderful guide. Finally somebody is putting to paper the necessary information we couldn't previously find all in one place. McCann-Beranger is naming the hard realities, while in the same breath challenging us to work with what strengths are remaining. Her use of language is very respectful, inclusive, and appropriate. For what families need, it's all here! When we are ready for more we are reminded to call the Alzheimer Society."

—Dr. Lise Hebert, PhD

A Caregiver's Guide

for Alzheimer *and* Related Diseases

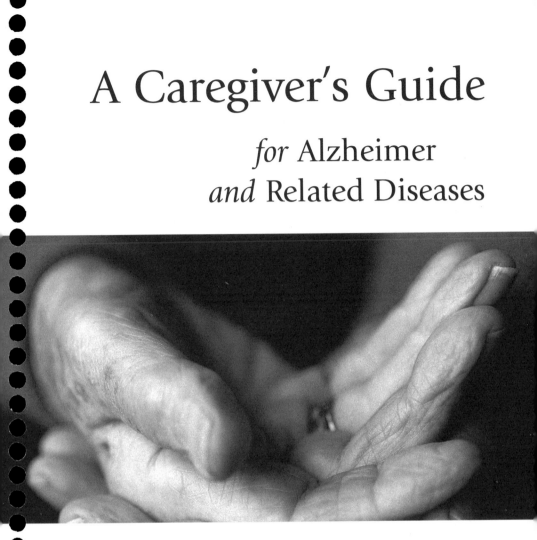

Judith McCann-Beranger

Société **Alzheimer** *Society*

A Caregiver's Guide for Alzheimer and Related Diseases
Second Edition © 2004 by Judith McCann-Beranger
ISBN 1-894838-11-4

A Caregiver's Guide for Alzheimer and Related Diseases
by Judith McCann-Beranger is also available in CD Format
ISBN 1-894838-12-2
To order: www.alzcaregiversguide.com

Originally published as
A Caregiver's Guide for Alzheimer Disease and Other Dementias
© June 2000 by Judith McCann-Beranger

For permission to reproduce parts of this *Guide* send a written request to:
Judith McCann-Beranger
Alzheimer Society of Prince Edward Island
166 Fitzroy Street, Charlottetown PE C1A 1S1

National Library of Canada Cataloguing in Publication

McCann-Beranger, Judith
A caregiver's guide for Alzheimer and related diseases / Judith McCann-Beranger.

Co-published by: The Alzheimer Society of Prince Edward Island.
Previously published under title: A caregiver's guide for Alzheimer disease and
other dementias.
Includes index.
ISBN 1-894838-11-4

1. Alzheimer's disease—Patients—Care. 2. Alzheimer's
disease—Popular works. I. Alzheimer Society of Prince Edward Island II. Title.

RC523.2.M33 2004   362.196'831   C2004-900609-6

The Acorn Press
P.O. Box 22024, Charlottetown, PE C1A 9J2
www.acornpresscanada.com

The Alzheimer Society of Prince Edward Island
166 Fitzroy Street, Charlottetown, PE C1A 1S1
www.alzheimer.ca

Cover design: Julie Scriver, Goose Lane Editions
Book design: Ron Walsh, Walsh Design
Illustrations: Dale McNevin
Printing: Transcontinental Prince Edward Island
Cover image: Veer

Note to readers:
For ease of style and reading, chapters will alternate the use
of male and female pronouns.

To Debbie Benczkowski
of the Alzheimer Society of Canada
for her dedication and outstanding contribution.

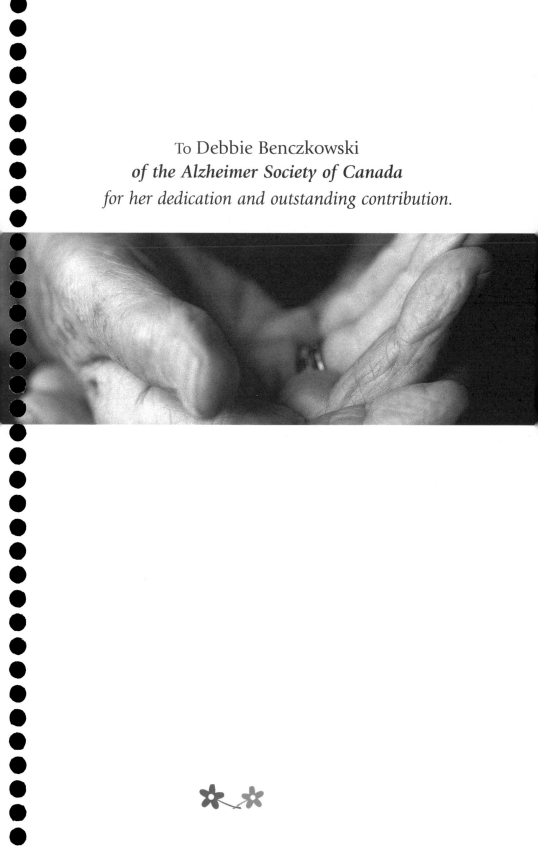

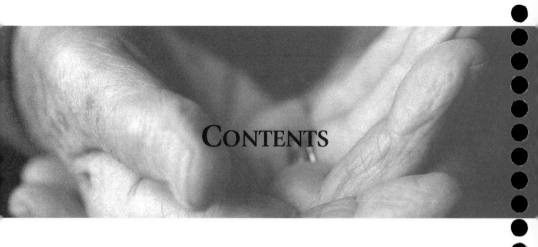

CONTENTS

Introduction   9

1. Diagnosis of Alzheimer Disease   11
- A Person Diagnosed with Alzheimer Disease
  Shares His Story 11
- What is Necessary for a Diagnosis of
  Alzheimer Disease? 14
- What Other Conditions Mimic the
  Symptoms of this Disease? 15
- What Should I Do if I Suspect
  Something is Wrong? 16
- The Challenge of this Progressive Disease 18

2. Alzheimer Disease   24
- What is Dementia? 24
- What is Alzheimer Disease? 24
- What is Happening in the Brain? 25

3. Progression of Alzheimer Disease   28
- The Early Signs 29
- Middle Progression 30
- Late Progression 31

4. Spirituality   32
- Why Consider Spiritual Activities? 33

- The Therapeutic Benefits of Spirituality 33
- Approaches to Spiritual Care 34

5. Meaningful Activities   36
- When Choosing Meaningful Activities 36
- Activities that Promote Quality of Life 37

6. Communication   39
- Your Approach 39
- When You Are Having Trouble
  Communicating 42
- Things to Avoid 43
- Hospitalization: What Families
  Need to Know 44
- Visiting 46
- Visiting the Doctor 48
- When You Are Concerned
  About Medical Care 48

7. Understanding Specific Behaviours   50
- Possible Explanations for Changes
  in Behaviour 51
- Defensive Behaviour 52
- Driving 55
- Restlessness 57
- Shadowing/Being Followed 58
- Sleep Problems 59
- Suspicion/Paranoia 60
- Wandering 62

8. Personal Care Activities   65
- Bathing 66
- Oral Hygiene 69
- Dressing 70
- Loss of Bladder/Bowel Control 72

9. Mealtimes   74
- The Table and Utensils 74
- Communication 75

- Agitation 75
- Tips About Food 76
- As the Disease Progresses 76
- If the Person Requires Meal Assistance 77

10. Treatments   79
- Aricept, Exelon, Reminyl 80
- Possible Side Effects 81
- Suggestions to Assist in Supervision of
  Treatments or Medications 81

11. Sexuality   83
- Myths & Misconceptions 83
- Sexual Functioning 86

12. Legal Concerns   90
- Wills/Living Wills 91
- Power of Attorney 92
- Establishment of a Trust 93

13. Safe Home Environments   95
- Safety 95
- Furniture/ Furnishings 97
- Bathroom 97
- Kitchen 98
- Bedroom 99

14. Late Progression of Alzheimer Disease   100
- Death and Dying 101
- The Grieving Process 102

15. Provincial Alzheimer Societies in Canada   105

16. Alzheimer Associations Around the World 107

Acknowledgements   109

Index   110

INTRODUCTION

As our population ages the world faces growing numbers of people affected by Alzheimer and related diseases. This *Guide* is intended to provide practical information for caregivers to help them adapt lifestyles and living environments that ensure a better quality of life and reduced stress levels for all involved. Informed caregivers are more likely to identify when they need time to recharge their batteries, and are also more likely to initiate activities that will enhance dignity and quality of life for the person with Alzheimer Disease.

Witnessing first-hand the decline of a family member is one of the most difficult emotional trials for any caregiver, family member, or friend. Reducing one's expectations, as the person becomes less and less able to respond and function, is a necessary adjustment. It is critical to accept that the person has a limited capacity to adapt or change his behaviour. Rather, caregivers must adapt their own behaviours and environments to the remaining abilities and strengths of the people for whom they are caring. The best way to determine if an approach will work is to try it, and adapt accordingly.

Adapting the environment is recognized as the most successful "treatment" for Alzheimer and related diseases.

The importance of keeping the person involved in normal daily activities cannot be overemphasized. Failure to stop the progression of this disease is no one's fault. Remember that your loving care and attention, along with environmental adaptations, will help maintain the person's remaining abilities as long as possible, and help preserve self-esteem. The Alzheimer Society can provide you with a list of programs, services, and resources that may help with your own unique situation.

I wish to thank the Alzheimer Society of Canada and the provincial Alzheimer Societies for use of their materials; the caregivers and the people living with Alzheimer Disease who provided input and advice and who are our greatest teachers; and all those who helped in reviewing this *Guide*. A very special thank you to my colleagues Gloria McIlveen, Wendy Schettler, Shelley Vaillancourt, and Gerard Murphy for going the extra mile with input, interest, and support. Thank you to Laurie Brinklow, whose gentle passion and expertise is invaluable. And finally to my husband, Greg, whose constant support and editing help truly makes this all possible.

—Judith McCann-Beranger
B.A., B.Ed., M.A., CCFE, Cert.C.Mediator

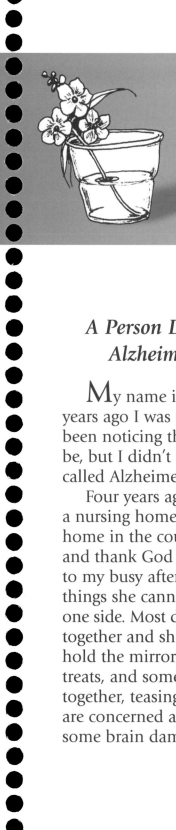

1. DIAGNOSIS OF ALZHEIMER DISEASE

A Person Diagnosed with Alzheimer Disease Shares His Story

My name is Fred Clarke and I am 84 years old. Two years ago I was diagnosed with Alzheimer Disease. I had been noticing that my memory was not like it used to be, but I didn't realize that it was bad enough to be called Alzheimer Disease.

Four years ago my wife had a stroke and had to go to a nursing home in Charlottetown. I moved in from our home in the country to be near her. I visit her every day, and thank God she is doing okay. I really look forward to my busy afternoons with my wife, helping her with things she cannot do for herself as she is paralyzed on one side. Most days when I get there I gather her make-up together and she puts it on with her good hand while I hold the mirror. I straighten up her room, keep her in treats, and sometimes do her nails. We enjoy laughing together, teasing each other and telling jokes. Lately we are concerned about her losing her appetite, she has some brain damage, but it could be a lot worse. We need each other very much and still enjoy being together.

I live at the Corrigan Lodge. It is very homelike and I am happy there. I still like to be independent, even though I get confused easily and can be very forgetful. I write notes to myself for reminders, and that really helps. I am getting by, and am grateful that I can still drive, even though I get lost easily. I keep out of traffic and don't do any night driving. I drive only when it is necessary and when the territory is familiar.

I am taking a medication, a drug that slows the progression of Alzheimer Disease. They say it only works for some, and I believe it is working for me. I had to be strong to keep fighting for this drug, as my health plan that funded it was cut off for a while. You have no idea how much stress I went through trying to get it back as part of my medical care. I had many sleepless nights. What a relief when I was told I would be covered for it again. I am hoping that I can stay on this drug long enough until something new comes along. As long as I can keep well I can visit my wife. I am satisfied, even if the only thing I am doing is slowing down the process. I am hopefully and anxiously waiting for a cure.

I am very thankful to God for what I do have. I feel very blessed in many ways. I have three wonderful sons and my wife. Even though she is not well I know she could be doing much worse. Being together with her gives me purpose. It makes me realize that even though there are many things I can't do, there are still so many things I can.

My greatest fear is getting lost, especially at night. Although it can happen in daylight, it seems worse if it happens at night. The confusion can happen at any time and it takes a little while to get back on track before it clears off. I am also afraid of becoming irritable. I think a lot and worry a lot when I go to bed. I know sometimes people can become very different than how they really are. I don't think that is happening to me yet, but I am afraid it might. Our sons are very good to us and I don't ever want to be a burden to them or anyone else.

One day I noticed in the paper that there was an Alzheimer Society Annual Meeting. I decided to attend, as I knew very little about what they did. I vaguely knew they offered something, but didn't think it would be of much value to me. Was I surprised! I don't remember anyone suggesting for me to go there, but I sure am glad I did. People really understand there. They are genuine. You know they want to help and they do. The staff are very capable and trustworthy. It's like we have known each other for a long time. Knowing they exist makes me feel like my luck has changed. Another good day!

I am sharing this because I believe it may help some-one else to have confidence in themselves and find out what is available out there to help them sooner than I did. We need to start talking about this disease and let people know that we are still able to do lots of things, and want to remain as independent as we can for as long as we can. I enjoy helping people and I plan to keep helping as long as I am able.

—**Fred Clarke**
Charlottetown, PEI

What is Necessary for a Diagnosis of Alzheimer Disease?

Although probability of an Alzheimer Diagnosis is accurate to 95 per cent through testing, actual confirmation of a diagnosis of Alzheimer Disease is possible only after death and an autopsy has been performed. Results may take many months. There is no single test to detect Alzheimer Disease. However, it is possible to have a clinical diagnosis based upon a comprehensive assessment, combined with a review of the complete history of current symptoms and previous functioning, and after eliminating all other possible causes of the symptoms. Recent research into diagnostic imaging is identifying the plaques and tangles in living tissue that may eventually lead to accurate diagnosis.

A valuable diagnostic tool for physicians is a carefully documented history, which should include the person's previous abilities, the appearance of symptoms such as forgetfulness, and any personality changes. Details of what family members observe are very important. They can provide significant information about the person's employment history, hobbies, and daily living patterns. This will help to illustrate the nature and extent of the changes taking place. Family members know best a person's "normal" changes and/or behaviours. They are the ones who are the closest in caring, and who know the importance of taking serious, concerns that are being expressed about memory or function. Keeping a daily diary that documents comments and changes is extremely valuable when talking to medical staff about the person living with Alzheimer or a related disease.

When visiting a physician or specialist, bring with you a complete list of medications—both prescription

14

and non-prescription. It can also be helpful to bring the containers as a back-up, to ensure proper names of medications and to check expiry dates. This is important, as drug reactions can sometimes mimic the disease, or worsen the symptoms.

A measure of cognitive functioning or thinking compares the person's ability to standardized normal scores in areas such as reasoning, judgement, orientation, general knowledge, and problem-solving. Such tests may be administered over a period of time to detect any gradual decline. A physical examination is necessary to detect other conditions that could be responsible for the symptoms. Laboratory tests may be necessary to rule out other disorders or infections that can mimic the disease. Further testing may include obtaining a psychiatric evaluation to test for conditions such as depression.

The purpose of these tests is primarily to rule out other possible, and perhaps treatable, causes of the person's symptoms. If treatable causes are found, the symptoms can often be reversed. Not every person requires all of these tests. Depending on the history of the person and what is found on a physical examination, the physician will decide on which tests are needed.

It is best to get the tests done when the problem is initially suspected. Some of these tests can be used for comparison if testing is repeated six to eight months later. Other tests may detect treatable problems such as drug reactions or infections.

What Other Conditions Mimic the Symptoms of this Disease?

- Brain tumours
- Abnormal thyroid function

- Infections
- Pernicious anemia
- Adverse drug reactions or alcohol abuse
- Certain hormonal imbalances
- Abnormalities in the spinal fluid system
  (e.g., hydrocephalus)
- Certain vitamin deficiencies (e.g., B Vitamins)
- Certain psychiatric conditions (e.g., depression)
- Unsuspected liver or kidney disease
- High blood calcium levels
- Multiple strokes
- Parkinson's Disease
- Acute physical illness
- Alcoholism
- Diabetes

My mom was very confused and often complained of dizziness. She started to think she was developing Alzheimer Disease. We asked our doctor to do whatever tests he could to find out what was wrong. Turns out Mom had low blood sugar and was diagnosed with diabetes. After the appropriate treatment, her confusion disappeared.

What Should I Do if I Suspect Something is Wrong?

- Express your concerns to your Family Physician
- Contact the Alzheimer Society
- Learn about the disease
- Plan for the future

A common dilemma for families is whether to tell the person about Alzheimer Disease once a diagnosis has been made. This is a decision that the family needs to discuss. Contact the Alzheimer Society for a copy of their *Ethical Guidelines on Communicating the Diagnosis*. Important points to consider:

- Knowing the diagnosis may put to rest the person's fear of not knowing what is wrong. Understanding the medical basis of the symptoms can alleviate guilt and frustration at not being able to do the usual things. Be on the alert for depression as it is also common with diagnosis.
- Knowing the diagnosis and prognosis, the person has the opportunity to discuss with family members and significant others what decisions she would like to make regarding the future. (When plans can be made together, such decisions do not rest as heavily on particular family members.) This allows all the family to play a part in respecting the person's final decisions and allows an opportunity to check with a lawyer and the Alzheimer Society for information about Health Care Directives early in the disease.
- Failure to talk about the disease may result in creating a communication barrier, or produce unnecessary guilt in family members.
- Sometimes the person will deny they have a disease that will get worse. The facts may seem too stressful and the diagnosis will not be discussed. Sometimes the caregiver may feel the same way.
- Support Groups are available in many places specifically for the person diagnosed. This provides an opportunity for people to share their wisdom and experiences of living with the disease. Contact the Alzheimer Society for contact numbers.

Early detection will encourage decision-making concerning business activities, retirement, financial planning, and future care. It will help the family to understand changes in the person, lessening feelings of frustration and anger. Having an early diagnosis ensures access to medications and the ability to take advantage of experimental drug-treatment trials. It allows for early participation in the planning and decision-making process, as well as providing the opportunity for attending support groups sooner rather than later.

The Challenge of this Progressive Disease

Damage to the brain caused by Alzheimer or related diseases makes people behave differently than they normally would. The person, no matter what the behaviour, deserves dignity, respect, and understanding from all those who care. People with the disease often cannot understand events happening around them and may have difficulty separating fact from fiction. It is very important not to take things personally.

The management of Alzheimer Disease can challenge the most skilled and experienced clinician. With no way to prevent or cure it, physicians or clinicians:

- may think that they have little to offer the person.
- can offer a thorough assessment and diagnosis.
- can offer symptomatic treatment, if appropriate.
- can give support and information to the person and their caregivers.
- can refer all involved to the Alzheimer Society.

It is important for family, friends, and neighbours to recognize and acknowledge the losses faced by the caregiver as well as the person living with this disease. Families and other caregivers can be more prepared to

18

help if they have a better understanding of the situation.
People with the disease:

- need to feel valued.
- face an uncertain future.
- may worry about becoming a burden to
  their families.
- need companionship.
- should strive to maintain an active and
  independent life.
- deserve to be treated with dignity and respect.

Caregivers:

- need to feel valued.
- may observe many changes in the person's behaviour.
- may not get the support of all family members.
- often feel alone and isolated from family
  and/or friends.
- consider it their duty to provide care.
- experience many role changes.
- will experience ongoing grief as they continually
  recognize new losses.
- may need assistance, but are often reluctant to
  ask. For example, grief counselling may help in
  dealing with ongoing losses.
- may sometimes need help in accessing support
  systems appropriate to their unique situation.
- may need help in accepting that any unfinished
  business with the person will likely go unresolved.
- find it helpful to have a quiet place or a special
  room, where they can rest, write in a journal, read,
  or just get away.
- find it helpful when they continue to encourage

independence and avoid the tendency to treat the person they are caring for like a child.

- find it helpful to keep a list of chores that can be shared as they recognize that family members or friends can be caregivers in different ways.
- experience stress that can affect overall health.
- need regular breaks from caregiving.
- may have a strong grief reaction if moving the person to nursing care (feelings of guilt, anxiety, and remorse).
- find it helpful to connect with the Alzheimer Society, learning as much as they can while using counselling, support groups, and other available services.

Caregivers should ensure they have updated personal and financial information filed in a secure place. It is important to know where all documents, investments, insurance policies, and keys are located. This also includes location and numbers of all bank accounts, any relevant tax information, driver's license, passport, Will, Power of Attorney, and social insurance and health card numbers. List all relevant phone numbers, including the lawyer, financial planner, and accountant.

Caring is incredibly demanding, and eventually will require around-the-clock care. For family caregivers, this commitment can last many years. Friends and neighbours are important sources of support for the family. Encourage caregivers to talk to the Alzheimer Society about difficult issues and to read their *Ways To Help* brochure. It talks about ways other family members, friends, and neighbours can help:

1. *Keep in touch*
A card, call, e-mail, or visit means a great deal. This disease has an impact on the whole family and everyone can benefit from your visits or calls. Continue to send cards

or letters, even if you don't get a reply. Continue to visit, even if the person does not recognize you. When visiting, choose a time that is best for the person, identify yourself, be patient and positive, allow time for a response, recall humorous experiences, and always include favourite stories.

2. Do little things—the little things are the big things
When cooking, make extra portions and drop off a meal (in a freezer-ready container). If you're on an errand, check with the caregiver to see if anything is needed. Surprise the caregiver with a special treat, such as a rented movie, library book, or gift certificate for a massage or dinner out.

3. Give the caregiver a break
Everyone needs a little personal time. Offer to stay with the person so the caregiver can have time out, run errands, attend a support group meeting, do a favourite activity, walk, listen to music, or attend a religious service. Even if the caregiver does not leave the house, this will provide personal time.

4. Help with a specific task
Often caregivers find it hard to ask for something specific. Have the family make a "to do" list of hard-to-get-done chores, such as laundry, yard work, or shopping. Decide what you can do, then dedicate some time to do the task on a regular basis.

5. Become informed
Learn about this disease and how it impacts on the family. For example, some people with the disease get disoriented at some point, and can become lost in their own neighbourhoods. One valuable resource is the *Safely Home—Alzheimer Wandering Registry*. The Registry is

designed to help those with the disease by registering them with local police agencies. Call the Alzheimer Society to register.

6. Provide a change of scenery
Plan an activity that gets the whole family out of the house. Make a reservation at a restaurant. Be sure to include the person being cared for, if the caregiver feels it is appropriate. You may wish to ask for a table with some privacy. You can invite the family to your house or to a nearby park for a picnic or a walk.

7. Learn to listen
Sometimes caregivers just need to talk with someone. Ask family members how they are doing and encourage them to share. Be available when the caregiver is free to talk. Try not to question or judge, but rather listen, support, and accept. You don't need to provide all the answers.

8. Take care of the caregiver
Caregivers need to eat well, exercise, and get enough rest so they can remain healthy. Encourage caregivers to take care of themselves. Pass along useful information and offer to attend a support group meeting with them.

9. Remember, all family members are affected
The person living with this disease will appreciate your visits, even if it doesn't appear that way. Hold a hand, give a hug, and treat the person the way you would want to be treated. Spouses, adult children, and even young children are all affected in different ways, and may experience stress from observing the difficulties of the family member. Be attentive.

10. Get involved

Help the caregiver fill out the Alzheimer Society's *Personal Care Book*. Consider volunteering or making a contribution to the Society. By choosing to actively do any of these things, you are providing help for today and hope for tomorrow.

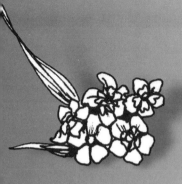

2. ALZHEIMER DISEASE

What is Dementia?

Dementia is not a disease, nor is it a diagnosis. Dementia is a general term used to describe a group of symptoms common to certain diseases or disorders. This group of symptoms includes the progressive loss of intellectual abilities, such as thinking, remembering, and reasoning. These symptoms are severe enough to interfere with a person's ability to function normally on a daily basis.

Alzheimer Disease is the most common form of dementia, accounting for approximately 64 per cent of all cases. Another form of dementia is vascular dementia, caused by multiple strokes (infarcts) in the brain. Some of the other diseases that produce dementia include Huntington's Disease, Pick's Disease, Creutzfeldt-Jacob Disease, Diffuse Lewy Body Disease, and Parkinson's Disease.

What is Alzheimer Disease?

Alzheimer Disease is a progressive, degenerative disease of the brain that destroys and damages brain cells.

It results in impaired memory, thinking, judgement, and behaviour. There is no known cause and no cure. It is not a part of normal aging.

Alzheimer Disease can last from a few years to over twenty years after symptoms are first recognized. The average duration is eight to twelve years. The disease manifests itself differently from person to person, even though there are many commonalities. Not everyone will exhibit the same problems at the same time in the disease. There is no one description of a "typical" person with Alzheimer Disease. Every case is unique in the severity and range of symptoms experienced. Symptoms depend on many factors, such as the stage of the disease, the person's pre-existing personality and coping strategies, environmental and social supports, and the presence of other diseases, such as diabetes, high blood pressure, or heart disease.

What is Happening in the Brain?

The brain is very complex and is made up of several distinct parts, each with its own function. It is composed of many different types of cells, but the primary functional unit is a cell called the neuron. All sensations, movements, thoughts, memories, and feelings are the result of signals that pass through neurons. Messages are passed between nerve cells (neurons) with the help of chemicals called neurotransmitters. During the course of Alzheimer Disease, many changes take place. These include:

- damaged nerve cells in the brain interrupt the passage of messages between the cells.
- at least one neurotransmitter (acetylcholine) is decreased. Other neurotransmitters may also be involved.

- the brain shrinks, reducing the surface area. The amount of surface area in the brain plays a part in how well a person can think and function. The spaces in the centre of the brain (the ventricles) become enlarged, leaving more empty spaces inside the brain.
- nerve cells develop changes that become the hallmarks of the disease. These changes include neuritic plaques and neurofibrillary tangles, which result in gradual loss of function.

Alzheimer Disease is a physical, neurological disease. The majority of the symptoms are cognitive and affect the ability to function. It is difficult for caregivers to accept some of the behavioural changes, especially when behaviours may change day-to-day. To some, it may appear as if the person is being purposefully troublesome. Alzheimer Disease damages the brain so that the person is no longer in control.

Family members and caregivers must reassess expectations of the person they are caring for, as there will be a gradual loss of ability to respond to situations or events. People with this disease will lose control of reactions and will not be able to explain why they are upset or why they acted so oddly. The progressive brain damage and resulting changes in behaviour cannot be stopped.

To cope successfully, caregivers must focus on remaining skills and abilities, not solely on the losses and changes. Adaptations to and cues in the environment, and in your approach, can enhance the remaining skills of the person. Initial signs of the progression are often subtle and may appear irregularly. The person often tries to cover up early changes. As a result, it may take some time for family members to realize that there is a serious problem. Early signs may include depression, forgetfulness, irritability, social withdrawal, decreased work performance, and perhaps behaviour that is out of character. A spouse may notice difficulty in the marital relationship and seek counselling. Co-workers may notice changes in work patterns.

Learning about the parts of the brain that are affected can be important, as recognizing weaknesses in one part of the brain allows caregivers to focus on strengths in another part of the brain. This new understanding of how different parts of the brain can be affected can help caregivers come to grips with behaviour fluctuations and changes. For example, when a part of the brain called the frontal lobe is affected, behaviour changes may include an inability to initiate tasks, socially unacceptable behaviour, and becoming easily distracted. This has implications for care as the person with dementia may not move spontaneously from one thing to another, and would not see particular behaviours as inappropriate.

If the temporal lobes are affected, behaviours may include an inability to recall what is seen, an inability to remember how to get around, or an inability to remember what was just said. Other areas affected are the limbic system, parietal lobes, and occipital lobe.

Just getting a cup of coffee creates a chain of events happening throughout various parts of the brain. One part of the brain tells you to start the process, another remembers where the coffee and filters are, a third part knows how to work the coffee maker, and so on. If one link in the chain of events is missing, the person will need assistance in completing the task. Once the ability is lost it is highly unlikely to be regained. Implications for the caregiver are great, as the person living with Alzheimer Disease may not remember what was just done or has just been told to him. Talk to your physician or the Alzheimer Society if you would like to learn more about this. The Alzheimer Society has an excellent video and reading material that explains this process very clearly.

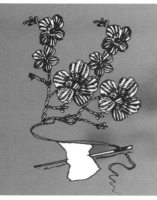

3. PROGRESSION OF ALZHEIMER DISEASE

Research into Alzheimer and related diseases has provided a general outline of how progression happens over time. Some health-care professionals use what is called a Global Deterioration Scale. This scale divides Alzheimer Disease into seven stages of decreasing ability. For the purposes of this *Guide*, we will explain the progression in three parts: early, middle, and late. Knowing what is likely to happen as the disease progresses will help those diagnosed and their caregivers to plan for the future. The duration of each stage, and the symptoms that appear, will be different with each person. The most common symptoms are described here and will serve as a general guideline to prepare families for future changes.

People living with Alzheimer or a related disease still have many abilities. They can continue to respond to sensory experiences (smell, sight, touch, taste, and sound), enjoy social situations, experience feelings and emotions, and find pleasure in humour and music. As people lose more skill function, it becomes increasingly important to emphasize what can still be done. This will maintain sense of self-worth and dignity. People diagnosed are adults, and deserve the respect and consideration of an adult.

A common challenge for families is coping with outbursts of temper or frustration. These displays of anger are often the result of the person's fear in realizing that something is wrong. Often anger can be directed towards oneself for not being able to do simple tasks that could once be done. This anger and frustration is sometimes transferred to someone close, such as the primary care-giver. The best advice is to remain calm and respond to the emotion, not the action, as reciprocating anger on your part will only increase the person's frustration.

The Early Signs

Reading is my favourite pastime. Now it seems impossible to retain anything of what I've read just minutes ago. This makes me feel horrified and helpless.

In the early progression of the disease incidences of common symptoms may only happen sporadically, but will increase in frequency as time progresses. Keeping a logbook or journal is very helpful for your own reference and also for bringing to appointments with the physician.

Symptoms may include:
- Mild communication difficulties (e.g., word-finding).
- Forgetfulness of recent events (this may be accompanied by denial of forgetfulness).
- Social withdrawal.
- Shorter attention span.
- Personality changes and "out-of-character" behaviours.
- Changes in approach to family, friends, and co-workers.
- Occasional confusion about the time or place.
- Inability to follow through with routine work patterns.
- Difficulty making decisions or finding routes

while driving a car.
- Difficulty in learning new things or remembering changes to an established routine.
- Poor judgement; less able to make sound decisions; orientation problems.
- Not reading as much as before and general decrease in ambition.
- Signs of depression (loss of appetite, poor sleep, physical complaints).
- Sporadic loss of ability to do complex, familiar daily activities, such as writing a cheque.

Middle Progression

One day my husband suggested that I check with the other guy about going for a walk. I didn't know whom he meant. A few nights later he got up from his chair in the living room, got his hat, and said it was time to go home as that other guy might not like him staying over. I realized then that the other guy was the one he saw in the mirror, and he no longer recognized himself or our home as his home.

Symptoms may include:
- Memory loss becoming more obvious; confusion about time and place.
- Increasing difficulty functioning in social situations.
- Loss of ambition; much more sitting and staring if left alone.
- Personality changes: paranoia, suspicion, insults, unpredictable behaviour, restlessness.
- Difficulty in recognizing others or self, particularly by name.
- Problems with communication.
- Difficulty with choosing proper clothing, starting or completing activities.

- Reasoning ability is severely impaired, affecting judgement.
- Problems with perception such as over-reaching for objects.
- Agnosia: inability to attach meaning to things one sees or hears. For example, the person may see the fork beside the plate, but not remember the purpose for the fork.
- Apraxia: the inability to carry out complex, purposeful movement, in spite of the physical ability to do so. For example, the person is still capable of getting dressed, but no longer understands how to do it.
- Loss of bladder/bowel control may begin.

Late Progression

By the end of the disease there was only about 5 per cent of my mother that I recognized. However, for her, the 5 per cent I was getting was 100 per cent of what she was able to give.

Symptoms may include:
- Complete dependence on others for care and safety.
- Inability to name family members and friends.
- Extreme confusion.
- Loss of ability to speak.
- Loss of bladder and/or bowel control.
- Difficulty eating independently, and may lose interest in food and/or have difficulty with chewing and swallowing.
- Loss of ability to walk.
- Becoming bedridden.
- Death due to the disease itself.

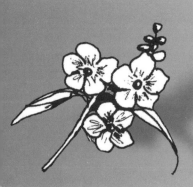

4. SPIRITUALITY

Spirituality is our unique response to life and is a much broader term than religion. By understanding all that it may represent for people, it is easier to assess and care for specific spiritual needs. Spirituality is an often overlooked and neglected need for people diagnosed with Alzheimer or a related disease. Embarking on a spiritual road in caring provides opportunities for expressing despair over this disease, resolving the past, and coming to terms with the frustrations of this disease. It also fosters hope, maintains dignity, and allows us to connect with others. It provides a foundation for the celebration of life. It helps to make meaning out of a situation, and to find a sense of inner peace.

Although organized religion can provide a structure for spirituality, people who consider themselves spiritual may or may not subscribe to any defined doctrine, or participate in any formalized rituals. Spirituality pertains to a sense of worth, meaning, and vitality; and connectedness to others, to life, and to the universe. It includes the expressions of one's spirit in a unique and dynamic process reflecting faith in something greater than oneself, thereby giving meaning and purpose. It is an integration of all human dimensions with a view to attaining inner harmony and self-actualization.

Why Consider Spiritual Activities?

- They can provide a wonderful sense of peace and hope.
- They provide an opportunity for reminiscing.
- They are a recognized source of support and reassurance.
- They provide an opportunity for spiritual and emotional expression.
- They are familiar activities and behaviours that provide comfort and connection with past experiences.
- They are an important part of the life experience of many; thus they are essential to holistic treatment.
- They represent a unique way of communicating, which can be very meaningful when standard communication fails.
- They are meaningful, adult activities.

The Therapeutic Benefits of Spirituality

- Making sense of a situation and assisting with the grieving process.
- Providing comfort, courage, and connectedness.
- Finding meaning or purpose in our day, our relationships, and our lives.
- Making sense of life and framing the past.
- Providing approval and acceptance.
- Encouraging acceptance of our mortality and that of our loved ones.

- Perceiving life in terms of the values we attribute to our experiences.
- Knowing we are loved, can give love, and hope.

Approaches to Spiritual Care

- Ensure music previously enjoyed is available. Favourite hymns can sometimes momentarily help people who no longer speak. When people are unable to speak, they are often still able to sing words to familiar songs.
- Share favourite prayers and Bible readings with the person.
- Take the person seriously, validating words and nonverbal cues.
- Speak with a gentle tone of voice.
- Provide opportunities for self-expression through art.
- Approach with a tender touch.
- Understand that the earliest long-term memories are the last to leave.
- Access memories through stories, pictures, meals, humour, religious symbols, and religious functions. This promotes reminiscence and creates endless connections to the spirit.
- Encourage participation in formal religion if that was important to the person. A special visit from clergy is valued and appreciated, and observing religious rituals still brings comfort.
- Have local clergy, Chaplains, or pastoral care workers visit regularly.
- Share the gifts found in nature and the beauty found in the seasons.

- Offer opportunities to stimulate the five senses to enable optimal interaction.
- Call your Alzheimer Society for other suggestions or referral.

Hope is the thing with feathers that perches in the soul,
And sings the tune without the words, and never stops at all.

—Emily Dickinson

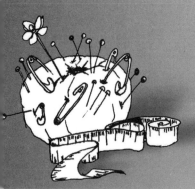

5. MEANINGFUL ACTIVITIES

Even though there are many losses associated with this disease, it is very important to recognize the strengths of the person you are caring for, and provide the opportunity for meaningful activities that promote dignity and respect. Activities include all the things we do, such as getting dressed, doing chores, playing games, planning visits with one or two people at a time, and even eating meals. The important thing is to make daily activities as meaningful as possible. Social situations involving even small amounts of excitement, laughter, and change may cause the person to become frightened, disoriented, or confused. Keeping active may help lessen changes in behaviour. Planned activities become meaningful to each person because they can represent who we are and what we're about. They can provide a sense of security, stability, fun, and togetherness.

When Choosing Meaningful Activities

- Concentrate on the person's strengths.
- Repeat activities that are successful and enjoyed.

36

- Choose a flexible activity that can be changed to suit the person's needs.
- Consider the person's former occupation or hobbies.
- Break the activity into steps.
- Emphasize the process of doing things, not the end result.
- Look for activities that make the person feel valued and productive. The person may prefer to just watch or help at first, and will join in later. Do not insist on participation. Just watching can be enjoyable for some.
- Avoid fast-moving activities that may cause anxiety or confusion.
- Avoid loud or noisy activities that may frighten or startle.
- Avoid activities where the person may fail.

Activities that Promote Quality of Life

Consider an activity a success if it brings enjoyment and helps the person feel needed and part of the family or group. Even if the activity seems boring to you, or it takes a long time to complete, it might be of great enjoyment to the person.

Recreational activities include:
- walks or drives
- listening to music, singing favourite songs, or playing instruments
- gardening
- visiting the park
- browsing through picture magazines
- going through old photo albums or scrapbooks

- cutting out pictures from old cards, calendars, or magazines to make collages
- playing games like crokinole, bean bags, and bowling
- dancing
- knitting
- reminiscing, using old props, coffee, and conversation
- visiting with young children
- visiting with a pet
- rekindling a favourite hobby

Helpful tasks include:
- setting or clearing the table
- dusting
- watering plants or gardening
- drying the dishes
- folding or ironing laundry
- winding yarn
- sorting thread or buttons
- folding grocery bags
- clipping coupons
- helping with food preparation by stirring or greasing the pan
- cutting out cookies for baking
- raking leaves
- washing the car
- cleaning windows
- light cleaning chores (even if only partially completed or need to be redone later)
- taking out the garbage
- caring for a pet (walking or feeding)

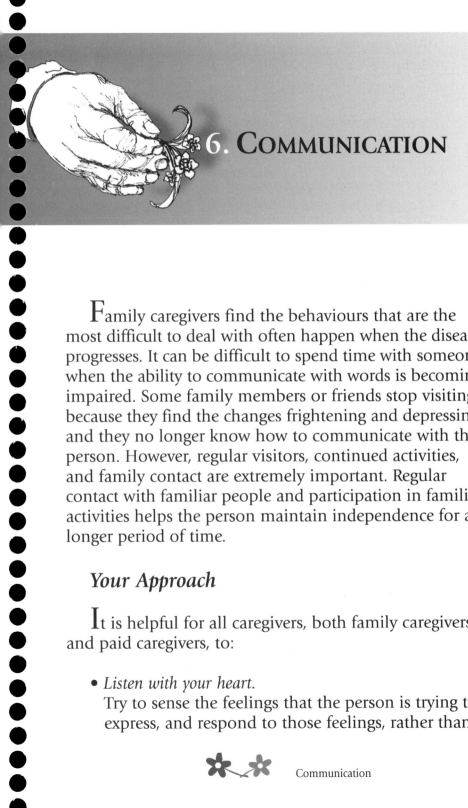

6. COMMUNICATION

Family caregivers find the behaviours that are the most difficult to deal with often happen when the disease progresses. It can be difficult to spend time with someone when the ability to communicate with words is becoming impaired. Some family members or friends stop visiting because they find the changes frightening and depressing, and they no longer know how to communicate with the person. However, regular visitors, continued activities, and family contact are extremely important. Regular contact with familiar people and participation in familiar activities helps the person maintain independence for a longer period of time.

Your Approach

It is helpful for all caregivers, both family caregivers and paid caregivers, to:

- *Listen with your heart.*
  Try to sense the feelings that the person is trying to express, and respond to those feelings, rather than

the words. Assume that all non-verbal expressions are attempts to communicate needs and/or feelings.

- *Think about how you are presenting yourself.*
  Are you tense? Frowning? People living with this disease are sensitive to non-verbal signals, such as facial expression, body language, and mood. If you are angry or tense, he is likely to respond by becoming angry, anxious, or annoyed.

- *Use a calm, gentle approach.*
  You set the mood for the conversation; your relaxed manner is contagious.

- *Use a non-demanding approach—try humour and/or cheerfulness.*
  Humour often helps caregivers through difficult moments. It will be more effective than ordering or demanding.

- *Use touch to help convey your message.*
  Touch can show caring when words are not understood. Some people may shy away from being touched, but most will find a gentle touch reassuring.

- *Reduce distractions.*
  People with dementia have difficulty screening out distractions in the environment, such as equipment noise, television, or other conversations. They will have trouble concentrating on what you are saying to them.

- *Maintain a normal, adult conversational structure.*
  Do not break down conversation into baby talk. Use normal sentence structure that is clear and simple. Provide openings in the conversation for the person to participate.

- *Begin conversations with orienting information.*
  Identify who you are, use the person's name often, and tell why you are there. This can reduce confusion and provide reassurance.

- *Face the person directly and maintain regular eye contact.*
  If you cannot get the person's attention, wait a few minutes and try again. Move slowly. Gently touch an arm or hand to gain attention, making sure to always approach from the front so as not to startle. Remember that as this disease progresses, there is loss of peripheral vision.
- *Make requests in ways that expect a positive response without giving orders.*
  For example, "The car is ready. Let's go to your doctor's appointment now."
- *Speak slowly and clearly. Ask questions requiring simple answers, such as yes or no.*
  Avoid open-ended questions. For example, instead of saying, "What would you like for breakfast?" simply ask, "Would you like eggs for breakfast?"
- *Allow plenty of time for a response.*
  Be comfortable with lengthy silences. It usually takes longer for the person to sort out what has been said and to organize a response.
- *Avoid questions with right or wrong answers. Seek opinions.*
  For example, ask the person if he likes the colour of the shirt, rather than what colour the shirt is.
- *Use concrete terms and familiar words.*
  As the disease progresses, people will lose the ability to understand abstract concepts and they interpret words and phrases literally. Avoid phrases and terms of speech such as, "You're pulling my leg." Provide missing words he is struggling for, unless you see this upsets him.
- *If repeating a question or statement, repeat exactly the same words.*
  The person needs time to process the information.

Changing the words may be confusing as it may appear that you are saying something entirely new.

- *Talk in a warm, relaxed, and pleasant manner.*
  Talk with a normal tone and pitch. Raising your voice may indicate to the person you are upset or angry, and may be confusing.
- *Demonstrate, visually, what you are saying.*
  If you are having difficulty making yourself understood, try using visual aids. For example, when asking, "Do you want to wear the red shirt?" hold up the red shirt so the person will know to what you are referring. Touch the chair when you are asking the person to sit down.
- *Make sure you are being understood.*
  Some people will not say they do not understand, and may cope by concealing poor memory or lack of understanding. Do not rely strictly on verbal responses for information, but use non-verbal clues as well.

When You Are Having Trouble Communicating

- *Listen actively and carefully to what the person is trying to say*
  If you don't understand, apologize and ask the person to repeat it. Let him know when you do understand.
- *Respond to the emotional tone of what is being said.*
  Recognize emotions such as anger or sadness in your response to a statement by saying, "You sound very angry." This acknowledges his emotional state, even if you cannot decipher the words.
- *Stay calm and be patient.*
  Remember that the person is not being purposefully difficult, and is probably even more frustrated than you are. Your calmness and patience will help create

a caring atmosphere that will encourage the person to keep trying.

Things to Avoid

- *Avoid entering an intimacy level that has not been earned.*
  Avoid using endearing terms like "sweetie," "dearie," or "honey," unless you are certain this does not bother the person. Family members who have developed pet names over the years best use these and other nicknames.
- *Avoid arguing with the person.*
  Remember that the person you are caring for no longer has the ability to be rational or logical to the same extent you do. The short-term memory is impaired, and it is often impossible to remember what just happened or to learn new things.
- *Avoid using a condescending tone.*
  A condescending tone is likely to provoke anger or humiliation, even if the words are not understood. Everyone deserves dignity and respect. Never use demeaning comments, such as, "How many times do I have to tell you?" or "You have asked me that five times this morning!"
- *Avoid questions that rely on a good memory.*
  Often our attempts to be sociable involve asking people about themselves. People with increasing memory loss may feel humiliated or angry if asked questions they can no longer answer. Try rephrasing. For example, instead of "Whose picture are you looking at?" say, "What a beautiful picture!"
- *Avoid relying strictly on the person's verbal response for information.*
  The person may say that he feels fine, or that he

does not know how to put on the shirt. However, this may just be a problem with verbal communication. Non-verbal behaviour may demonstrate that he is, in fact, in pain, or that he can still put on the shirt.

- *Avoid talking about the person as if he wasn't present.* It is easy to fall into the habit of talking in front of people when they can no longer communicate well. It is impossible to know how much someone understands, and this may vary from moment to moment. Always try to include the person in the conversation.

Hospitalization: What Families Need to Know

Family members know the person they are caring for better than anyone; your involvement can do much to facilitate care and treatment. It is important to remember that people affected with Alzheimer and related diseases get other illnesses. If your family member requires other medical treatment, explore care options with the attending physician. In some situations, you may want to inquire if treatment can be administered on an out-patient basis, at home by a visiting nurse, or from a facility that is better equipped to deal with people who are confused and sometimes disoriented. In most cases these options are less threatening and more comforting for the person. When hospitalized, the person may become increasingly confused and disoriented. This is due primarily to a change of environment, medications, and/or comfort zone. For medical conditions that can only be effectively treated in hospital, consider the following:

44

- A hospital social worker is available to help with questions, support, and counselling.
- Most hospitals were not designed to care for people who may wander around and become lost and disoriented. Serious security concerns arise when a patient is immobilized on a medical or surgical unit, and each nurse has many others to care for at the same time. People who are confused often cannot receive the one-on-one, constant care they require. A person who wanders away can disappear in minutes.
- Staff at the hospital are trained and ready to address the person's medical problems, but may not be trained to provide the additional special care required due to this particular disease.
- It is not realistic to expect all hospital staff to be able to immediately identify all those people who have Alzheimer or a related disease on their unit. Often people can cover their problem with conversation and social skills, thus appearing quite normal.
- It is very important that family members, friends, or other caregivers provide as much information as possible to the hospital doctors and nurses who will be providing care. If staff are made aware, they can make greater efforts to ensure the environment meets the safety, comfort, and dignity needs of the person. Connect with the head nurse and find out the best place to bring your comments and/or concerns.
- Family members and friends who are able to provide assistance by spending time with the person are encouraged to do so. The most ideal care that a person can receive is from someone close to him who understands his capabilities, strengths, and limitations; likes and dislikes; fears and anxieties; and who is capable of advocating on his behalf. If

family members are not available to provide care, then a trained person or respite worker could be hired as needed.

- A conference with the physician, nurse, and caregivers can be helpful during the hospital stay. If this opportunity is not provided, put in a request. This can help identify problems while planning care management for the return home. Current medications can be reviewed and discussed. The need for assistance of home care may also be determined.

Be aware of what hospitals can and cannot provide. Ask questions. Provide them with a completed *Personal Care Book* available from the Alzheimer Society. This will give important details, likes, dislikes, and stories about the person. Inquire as to whether the people who will be providing the care have training in Alzheimer and related diseases. Open communication with all who are providing care is critical. Do everything you can to ensure that the person's security, dignity, and safety needs are addressed.

Visiting

It is important for other family members, friends, and neighbours to keep visiting the person no matter where they are in the progression of the disease. Even when people have lived with the disease a long time and we are not sure they know who we are, it is important to stay connected. This is supportive to both the caregiver and to the person living with the disease.

- Arrange a suitable time for the visit.
- Be relaxed and don't give the appearance of being in a hurry.

- Speak quietly and slowly and in simple sentences, never rushing.
- Walking around with the person is a good way to get acquainted. Going arm in arm can direct the progress and give a sense of warmth and caring. Talk about things you know they enjoy.
- Chat about the wall colours or the plants or the bird in the cage or the fish in the tank. Talk about everyday happenings, the seasons, flowers in the garden, and children or grandchildren. Know favourite stories.
- Take a picture or photograph album with you.
- If the person cannot talk, give a gentle greeting using his name.
- The sound of your voice and touch of your hand are the best gifts.
- Garbled speech and tears are common in some people. Don't panic. Continue to talk in a soothing voice.
- Sit near and talk directly, making eye contact. If you feel comfortable, touch or hold the person's hand while conversing.
- Be patient; wait for a response. Look interested. Just holding hands may be response enough.
- Ten or fifteen minutes may sometimes be long enough for a first visit.
- Have a laugh together over a picture you have brought from a paper or magazine, and give a hug when you leave.
- Remember the caregiver. Offer to run errands or provide help.
- Encourage the caregiver to take a break from care giving. A few days away or a couple of weeks' vacation will do wonders in helping the caregiver

recharge his batteries.
- Never stop visiting and never believe your visits are fruitless.

Visiting the Doctor

Communicating clearly with your physician is crucial. Building this relationship to include regular, scheduled visits with enough time will ensure a better quality of life for everyone concerned. If you are not pleased with something happening during your visits, talk with the doctor.

- Consider the best time of day for you.
- Keep a regular journal, making points about the health of the person you are caring for, as well as your own health. Include symptoms experienced by the person and what is happening when the symptoms occur. Include medications taken and times they are taken, as well as any reactions. Bring these notes to the appointment with you.
- Keep a list of questions to ask the doctor and be prepared for a follow-up visit if time is limited.
- If you want your time to listen and concentrate, bring someone along to take notes. Find out where you can get more information to read up on concerns.

When You Are Concerned About Medical Care

The College of Physicians and Surgeons tries to make sure that you get the best medical care possible by allowing only medical doctors licensed by the College to practice. If you are concerned about the care your family member has been receiving from your medical doctor, talk to him about it. He will appreciate your input. If this proves unsuccessful, try a second opinion. The Medical Society in your province or state will also provide advice. If all attempts prove fruitless, you can write to the College. The Alzheimer Society can provide you with the address of the Registrar of the College of Physicians and Surgeons.

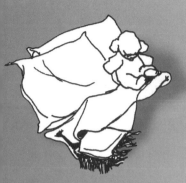

7. UNDERSTANDING SPECIFIC BEHAVIOURS

As the disease progresses, a person's confusion will increase. This could result in events such as mistakenly throwing out the groceries, eating the toothpaste, or putting the laundry in the fridge. Behaviours that can lead to problems may appear. The presence of these behaviours will vary from person to person, and will change as the disease progresses.

Behaviours are not only different from person to person, but even day to day for the same person. Someone may be able to use the washroom independently in the morning, but may require assistance in the evening. Changes in functioning may be due to how the person is feeling, medications, illness, fever, what activities or visitors the day included, or the person's energy level. During some parts of the day a person may have more energy than at other times, and therefore may be able to do more. When energy is low, defensive behaviours may appear more difficult as the person finds the environment increasingly confusing.

It is possible to reduce day-to-day frustrations by using certain techniques to cope with defensive behaviours, thereby improving the quality of life for both yourself and the person for whom you are caring. A golden rule cited by many caregivers is to establish consistent routines and a regular rhythm of familiar household events. The person is struggling to maintain an understanding of what is going on in the environment, and frequent changes or routines will only increase helplessness.

Possible Explanations for Changes in Behavior

- *Physical/Emotional Well-Being of the Person*
  Side effects of medication, physical illness or discomfort, depression or fatigue may trigger defensive behaviours. Always monitor specific behaviours and consult the person's physician.
- *Environmental Causes*
  Too many distractions or activities happening, an unfamiliar environment, or no cues to orient the person to the new environment may cause confusion, panic, and agitation. Loss of light in the environment can increase confusion.
- *Task-Related Causes*
  Tasks may be too complicated, or unfamiliar. Activities may have to be broken down into small steps, and given to the person one step at a time.
- *Problems in communication can also lead to defensive behaviours*
  When people are not feeling heard or understood, feelings such as frustration, helplessness, anger, impatience, and sadness arise, and may sometimes lead to changes in behaviour. The damage to the brain caused by the disease makes people behave differently than they would normally, sometimes appearing stubborn, mean, suspicious, or ungrateful.

At times the defensive behaviour is beyond rational explanation, but remember that the person is still an adult deserving of dignified treatment at all times.

Defensive Behaviour

People with this disease tend to react emotionally to events. When tired, uncomfortable, frightened, or confused, they may express these feelings through anger. These are not deliberate actions to upset you. If nothing is done to reduce or change this response, emotions can escalate.

Understanding and Preventing Defensive Behaviours

- Learn and understand as much as you can about the disease process.
- Understand unusual behaviours such as the person trying to communicate unmet needs.
- Watch for warning signs of distress or anger, and take preventive actions immediately.
- Simplify the environment by reducing or eliminating excess noise, such as turning off the TV, regulating the number of people coming and going, and reducing household clutter.
- Alternate quiet times with more active periods.
- Plan outings and activities when the person is fully rested.
- Do not make frequent changes around the household.
- Keep your daily routine as consistent as possible.
- Introduce any necessary changes gradually, e.g., a new caregiver assistant should be introduced slowly, allowing time for adjustment.
- Regular exercise will help to reduce stress. Try walking or dancing.

- Should you ever require assistance, be sure to have an emergency plan of action in place, including telephone numbers.

Strategies That May Help

It is helpful to take time to think about your own ways of dealing with emotional events. How would you act if you felt afraid, anxious, frustrated, angry, happy, or sad? How would you demonstrate these feelings if you couldn't express yourself in the usual ways? Observe the person and the environment.

- Keep a journal detailing each incident—where it happened, who was present, what you were doing, the time of day, etc. Caregivers can often find a pattern and discover preventive techniques as a result.
- Approach from the front, maintaining a calm reassuring manner and tone of voice.
- Make sure the person is comfortable. Check that clothes are not too tight, that the temperature is not too hot/cold, or if there is a need to go to the bathroom.
- Remove the person from the stressful situation, gently guiding away from the environment while speaking in a calm, reassuring voice.
- If the person is very upset, put something in her hand, which, if thrown, will not hurt anyone (e.g., facecloth). This distracts and provides something different on which to focus .
- Music, massage, or quiet readings may have a calming effect.
- Use gentle touch to calm a person. Holding hands and hugging may offer reassurance to some people, but may be perceived as restraining to others.

- Use distractions, such as looking at a photo album or having a snack.

It is not uncommon for the person to emotionally and/or physically lash out at those who are the closest—even with the most loving caregiver. Generally, this is hard to explain or understand, but there is usually a reason for such behaviour. Stay calm. Use a soft, reassuring voice and a soothing touch. Distraction often works best. Try to draw attention to something familiar. The person will often forget what took place and why she was angry. However, such episodes are very upsetting to the caregiver, and not easily forgotten. Accept the fact that it is not being done on purpose. It is possible that the aggressiveness is self-directed and that the person is upset with herself.

If you think your physical safety is threatened, consider the following:
- Be aware of what you may be communicating non-verbally.
- Avoid trying to gain control of the issue. Let it go.
- Stand out of reach of the person, and identify yourself to the person.
- Clear the area of potentially dangerous objects.
- Leave the scene to prevent injury, if necessary.
- Call for help. Call neighbours, family members, friends, or your physician.
- Call the police as a last resort.

After an episode has passed, do not remind the person of the incident. It will probably soon be forgotten. Consider what can be changed to avoid an episode from recurring. Have an emergency plan in mind and discuss it with other members of the household, friends, and/or neighbours.

Driving

Early diagnosis doesn't automatically mean a person has to stop driving. However, the progression of the disease will eventually cause safety issues in driving. Family members need to be aware when it is no longer safe. Sometimes the person will recognize that it is time to make the decision to no longer drive, but often the family must take the necessary and difficult steps to see that the person no longer drives.

Strategies that may help:
- Compensate by providing access to transportation for leisure as well as necessary appointments.
- Disable the car—removing the battery is sometimes helpful if there are no other drivers.
- Ask your physician to talk to the person about no longer driving.
- Discuss this decision with the person in the hope that she will understand.
- Keep the car and car keys out of sight.
- Never leave the person unattended in a car. She may become frightened about being left alone, could wander away, release the emergency brake, or fiddle with the gearshift.

Getting Into the Car
Difficulty often arises when getting into the car. As the disease progresses, perceptual problems may develop, often making it difficult for the person to recognize differing depths. As confusion increases, the once logical

and habitual steps necessary to get into and out of a car are forgotten.

A recommended reading, *Therapeutic Caregiving* by Barbara Bridges, talks about many ways that may help to ensure the safety and comfort of the person travelling with you. The following steps may help:

- Park your car on a flat surface a fair distance from the curb. Leave enough room for the person to step onto the street and to be able to turn to sit.
- Move the front seat back as far as possible so there is lots of room to move. The front seat of the car is often more accessible than the rear seats.
- Clothing may stick to car seats made of velour or cloth. Try covering the car seat with more slippery material, such as a sheet of plastic, to ease movement and shifting. Open the front door first; turn the person around so that her back is facing the inside of the car. Hold the person's hands in yours, or place her left hand on the door and her right hand on the back of the door frame. Back the person up until the backs of her legs are touching the car seat.
- Ensure the person's feet are outside the car and firmly on the ground; guide the person to sit sideways on the seat; protect the head.
- Once seated, direct the person to pull in her left leg, and then the right. Once legs are inside, the person can shift or swivel around to face the front of the car. Direct the person to scoot her bottom towards the back of the seat.
- Buckle up. If the person attempts to remove the seatbelt while driving, turn the seatbelt inside out so that the buckle is not easily accessible.
- Lock the door.

Restlessness

People with Alzheimer and related diseases depend upon cues in the environment. As sunlight decreases, cues decrease and people may go through a period of increased restlessness, confusion, and agitation. Restlessness in the late afternoon and early evening has been referred to as sundowning, "after the sun goes down." This may be due to various reasons, including the person being tired or not being active enough during the day. She may be following past habits or routines, such as going home after work, or preparing a meal. This could also be due to the loss of vitamin D. The theories are varied and many. A person may demonstrate restlessness or tiredness by continuous walking or pacing. It is usually more severe in unfamiliar situations, such as waiting in a doctor's office.

Strategies that may help:
- Use distraction, such as a walk, or putting on music. Television is generally not a good idea for distraction. A person may confuse the fiction with reality and become more confused and agitated.
- If at an appointment, bring along a photo album or favourite magazine to go through together. Try to arrange appointments for the morning, if that is when the person is at her best.
- Create an area where the person can pace safely.
- A rocking chair or exercise bike may release excess energy.
- Involve the person in regular exercise.
- Do not announce planned activities too far in advance, as the person may become restless due to uncertainty about when she must leave or begin the activity.

- Eliminate beverages containing caffeine, particularly before bedtime.
- Plan other activities, such as a household chore or a walk.
- Include the person in meal preparation that follows habits from the past.
- Close the curtains before dark to shut out the nightfall and window glare.
- Turn on lots of lights to brighten the environment and combat shadows. Some people benefit from light therapy, especially in winter months.
- Try to be rested for better coping at the most agitated time of the day.
- Minimize noise, confusion, and numbers of people around during the most agitated time of the day.
- Ensure plenty of exercise (walks, dancing, and swimming) during the day.

Shadowing/Being Followed

People with dementia are more prone to fear and anxiety as they lose their sense of the familiar. They are anxious about whether a caregiver who leaves the room will return, or who will pick them up from an appointment. This "fear" can result in the person shadowing the caregiver, following her everywhere. The person with Alzheimer Disease becomes very attached to the one constant in life: the primary caregiver.

Strategies that may help:
- Reassure the person where you are and what you are doing.
- Plan activities you can do together, such as peeling vegetables, or drying dishes.

- Arrange a break from caregiving for yourself, as this behaviour can be very tiring and you will need a respite.

Sleep Problems

This is a difficult problem for caregivers. Some people with Alzheimer or related disease do not sleep well at night and may wander around the home, turning on lights or the stove. They may even find their way outside.

Strategies that may help:
- Keep on nightlights leading to the bathroom —this provides a cue and security.
- Arrange for a medical check-up to identify a possible medical cause for the sleep problems, including an evaluation for depression.
- For some, a bedside radio tuned softly to favourite music is helpful.
- Read to the person with dementia from a source with which she is familiar and has previously enjoyed.
- Check to make sure the person is comfortable, not hot, cold, hungry, or has to use the bathroom.
- Give a backrub or massage legs at bedtime.
- Allow the person to sleep on a couch or in an armchair if she refuses to get into bed.
- Suggest a drink of warm milk.
- Offer a bedtime snack.
- Avoid caffeine and other stimulants (tea, coffee, chocolate, cola drinks) in the evening.
- Make sure the person goes to the bathroom before going to bed.
- Have the person spend less time in bed, by getting

up earlier in the morning, or cutting down on daytime naps.

- Set a reasonable bedtime. If a person goes to bed at 8:00 in the evening, it may not be unusual to wake up at 3:00 in the morning.
- Maintain a bedtime and waking routine, and continue any bedtime rituals from the past (e.g., a glass of milk before bed, or music on the radio at bedtime).
- Plan for adequate exercise during the day.
- Avoid upsetting activities, such as bathing in the late afternoon or evening, unless this has been part of the person's past routine and offers comfort. This is when the person should be winding down.
- Avoid laying out clothes for the next day or talking about the next day's activities. This may be confusing and give a "wake-up" signal.
- Avoid reliance on sleeping medication, as it can lead to other problems.
- Make the house safe for the person to wander alone at night, by removing knobs on the stove or having an electrician install a safety switch. Place locks on doors out of sight or reach.
- The caregiver needs to plan ways to compensate for loss of sleep. A respite program can be very helpful. Talk to someone at the Alzheimer Society for ideas and suggestions.

Suspicion/Paranoia

The person with dementia may begin to accuse people close to her of various things. The person cannot understand events happening around her. Judgement is impaired due to damage to the brain, making it difficult to separate fact from fiction. Items such as eyeglasses and jewellery may be misplaced. When unable to locate the missing item, she may accuse someone else of stealing the article. Explanations or attempts to reason may only produce further suspicion and anger.

Strategies that may help:
- Offer to help look for misplaced items, but do not scold the person for losing or hiding things. If possible, keep a spare set of those items that are frequently missed, and learn where favourite hiding places are.
- Explain potentially frightening misinterpretations: "That loud noise is the train passing by."
- Do not directly disagree with a false idea by arguing. Instead, identify with the emotion being expressed, e.g., "You sound lonely," then attempt distraction, e.g., "Let's go for a walk."
- Use familiar distractions: music, exercise, card-playing, photo albums, playing with pets.
- Talk about the missing object. For example, Mrs. Brown can't find the picture of her mother. Reply by stating how she must miss her mother, and remind her of the great cookies and bread she used to make all the time.
- Have vision and hearing checked.
- Change the environment as little as possible.
- Maintain daily routines such as meal and bedtime rituals. Routines give structure and a sense of the familiar to the person who lives in an increasingly unfamiliar world. Even a few simple daily routines can help provide a sense of security.
- Provide opportunities for the person to feel in control.
- For severe paranoia, contact your physician.

A person who is increasingly confused awakens each day in unfamiliar surroundings, having forgotten her environment and the trusted people in it. It is understandable that she may become suspicious. Do not take accusations personally. Remember that personality changes are a result of the disease, and this person would not behave in this manner if she were well.

Wandering

Many people with dementia like to keep moving. They may be focused on going somewhere or doing something, then forget where they are. As the person becomes more confused about the environment and people around her, she may continue to wander, hoping to find someone or something familiar, such as her childhood home. The person may just walk away from a situation, very happy to continue walking alone, without a thought as to how to get back home later. The rhythmic, repetitive action of the walking itself is probably comforting. Talk to the Alzheimer Society about any concerns you may have, and consider registering the person you are caring for on the *Safely Home Registry*.

Strategies that may help:
- Check to see if the person is hungry, needs to use the bathroom, or is in pain.
- Allow the person to walk freely if the environment is safe. Consider setting up a safe walking space in or near the home, and ask neighbours to keep alert.
- Decrease noise levels and the number of people interacting with the person at one time.
- Remove items from sight that may trigger a desire to go out, e.g., boots, coats.

- Distract with food, conversation, or activity.
- Involve the person in the household routine, e.g., cleaning, and folding laundry.
- If the person cannot be gently dissuaded from leaving, walk with her. Gradually change the course, without saying so, and begin to walk towards home. Walking or other exercise often reduces the frequency and severity of wandering behaviour.
- Have the person go for a medical check-up, especially if exhibiting unusual behaviour.
- Keep familiar objects, furniture, and pictures in the surroundings to increase a sense of security.
- Help direct the person with clearly labelled rooms. For example, put a picture of a toilet on the bathroom door.
- Observe the time of day the walking usually begins or whether there are certain events that tend to precipitate wandering. Then try scheduling activities at these times to reduce the activity if it is problematic.
- Provide frequent reassurance to the person that you are there to provide for her care.
- Ask for help. For example: "Would you help me with the dishes?"
- Place nightlights throughout the house.
- Place locks out of sight or reach, such as at the bottom or top of the door. Place warning bells above doors leading to the outside to signal that someone is leaving the house.
- Investigate monitoring systems available for home environments.
- Notify close friends and neighbours to contact you should the person be seen wandering.
- Sew name and address tapes on clothing. Ensure the person always has identification.

- Don't fix squeaky doors or floorboards, as this can serve as an alert signal for wandering.
- Keep a current photograph of the person on hand.

Wandering results from urges or restlessness that the person cannot control. Losing her way in the dark, forgetting where she is going or why, can be very frightening to a person whose memory, judgement, and reasoning are impaired. If a person does go missing, try not to panic. Wait a few minutes before starting a neighbourhood search or calling the police. Sometimes the person will just go to the end of the street and back. Have a quick scan of your street and yard.

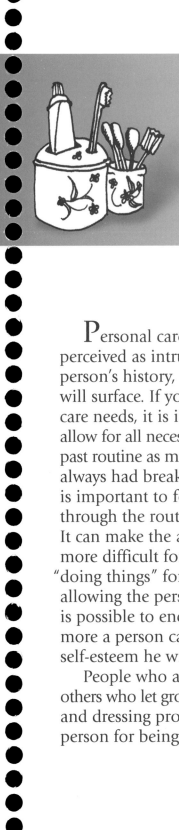

8. Personal Care Activities

Personal care is an intimate time and can often be perceived as intrusive. If there are any trauma stories in a person's history, this will likely be the time when they will surface. If you are assisting someone with personal care needs, it is important to block off plenty of time to allow for all necessary activities while following the person's past routine as much as possible. For example, if the person always had breakfast in his robe and then got dressed, it is important to follow that same routine. Do not rush through the routine of bathing and shaving, or dressing. It can make the activity traumatic and unpleasant, and more difficult for the caregiver. It may be hard to resist "doing things" for someone because he may be slow. By allowing the person to participate in his personal care, it is possible to encourage independence and dignity. The more a person can accomplish for himself, the more self-esteem he will maintain.

People who are neat and clean usually feel better than others who let grooming habits go. Activities such as bathing and dressing provide opportunities to acknowledge the person for being clean and attractive. Bath time is also a good time to watch for any skin infections or problems, including the need for foot care. Several of the following suggestions can be applied to many different activities. Make a note of the ones that work best in your situation, and try them under different circumstances.

Bathing

The towel bath, a gentle sponge bath method, is an alternative for those who refuse bathing. Taking a full bath is a complex activity involving many steps. It can be very confusing and overwhelming for someone who does not remember doing it before. It is fairly common for people to resist the activity of bathing during some point in the disease. Resistance is based on fear and anxiety, not a desire to remain unclean. Some of the following suggestions will help caregivers should they encounter problems.

- *Could it be a perceptual problem?*
  People will experience problems with perception. The ability to judge distance may be impaired. In the case of taking a bath, the person may not be able to judge the depth of the tub just by looking at it. To him, it may appear extremely deep and frightening. A contrasting, non-slip mat on the bottom of the tub will indicate where the tub ends, and light bubbles on the surface of the water will show where the water begins. Placing a contrasting, damp towel over the edge of the tub will help define the edge of the tub.

- *Break the activity into several smaller steps*
  Write down all of the individual steps involved with taking a bath or shower. If the person seems

overwhelmed with all that is involved in bathing, try introducing the person to one step at a time, rather than presenting the activity as a whole. Perhaps start with undressing, then into the tub, sitting down, then using the soap and washcloth.

- *Know the person*
  - Fill out the *Personal Care Book* available from the Alzheimer Society. Should hospitalization or assistance from other caregivers be required, this book will help others know past bathing routines.
  - Be familiar with the regular bathing routines of the person—does he prefer a tub bath, a shower, or sponge bath.
  - Know if morning, noon, or night was the bathing routine, and how often during the week this was done.
  - Notice whether the person has a preference for a male or female helping in his care.

- *Set the mood*
  - Use a calm, personal, gentle manner.
  - Create a feeling of privacy.
  - Play soft music in the background to create a calming and relaxing atmosphere, or sing a song you know the person enjoys.
  - Use scented soaps and soft, colourful towels and robes to make the bath a pleasant, sensory experience.

- *Prepare the bathroom*
  - Make sure the bathroom is warm and inviting.
  - Collect all necessities and place within easy reach, including towel, soap, washcloth, skin lotion, supplies for mouth/tooth care, etc. Give items in order of use to help the person do what he can by himself.

- Remove bathroom articles not necessary for the bath, as they can distract the person from the task at hand, and will interfere with his ability to concentrate on what he is doing.
- Provide adequate lighting.

- *Getting started*
  - First, spend a few moments sitting and socializing to develop a sense of comfort and trust.
  - Start with an invitation, "I have a nice warm bath ready for you—let's go this way."
  - Explain what you are going to do during each step. The person may be easily startled or upset by a sudden movement or an unexpected procedure.
  - Be sure that all the body is washed to avoid rashes or skin infections.
  - Wrap a towel around the shoulders of the person sitting in the tub and fasten with a clothespin if he feels embarrassed about being undressed. It is important to respect the person's privacy and dignity.
  - Start by gently offering the warm, wet facecloth and placing it in the person's hand. He may automatically start to bathe. Do not start by washing the face as this may startle and frighten the person.

- *Resistance*
  - If the person resists being bathed, distract him for a moment and then try again with gentle persuasion. Do not attempt to use force. This may result in frightening the person and the possibility of him striking out at you.
  - Give a reason for bathing, e.g., going to church or to the doctor; your hair is dirty; company is coming.

- Try giving the person a washcloth to hold or some-thing safe to fiddle with for distraction while bathing.
- Offer a mint or candy to preoccupy the person.
- A person may resist bathing because of embarrassment with your presence. Consider having Home Care or other support services in two or three times a week for this purpose.
- If the person had been accustomed to bathing on Saturday, try saying two or three times a week, "It's Saturday, time to take a bath."
- Try offering a choice of alternative times for a bath.
- Reduce the number of baths to a minimum.
- Come back later when the person's mood is better.

- *Safety*
  - Ensure water temperature is not too hot and that taps cannot easily and/or accidentally be turned to extreme temperatures.
  - Handrails, detachable hand-held showerheads, and other aids are available, and can make bathing much easier.
  - Provide non-slip secure footing in the tub or shower.
  - If showers are the custom, try showering with the person. Sometimes this is the simplest solution, although not all caregivers are in a position to do this.
  - If the person tires easily, have a bath bench handy or already in the tub to use during the bath/shower.

Oral Hygiene

- Upon diagnosis, get a complete dental check-up and attend to any problems right away. It will only get more difficult and frightening for the person if it is delayed.

- Schedule dental appointments in the morning, when the person is often at his best. Alert the receptionist in order to eliminate a long wait in the reception room. Bring along a favourite magazine, photo album, or something familiar.
- Make sure teeth are brushed. If needed, initiate the activity of brushing by placing the toothbrush with paste in the person's hand and gently guide to the mouth.
- Use special rinses after brushing. Make sure it is a substance that is not harmful if accidentally swallowed.
- The person may resist by biting down on the brush, closing the mouth tightly, or spitting out the toothpaste. (Toothpaste without foam tends to work best.) Never pry the brush from between the teeth. Wait until the jaws relax and try again. Try humour and a non-demanding approach. Get advice from your dental professional.
- Be patient. Speak gently and quietly; explain each move, and how important it is to take good care of the teeth.
- Try brushing your teeth at the same time. This will help the person understand what to do.
- If the person wears dentures, and you can afford it, consider purchasing a spare set. These can be stored in a safe place in case the person misplaces or loses the first set.

Dressing

Everyone likes to look his best. Even if the person is unaware of his appearance, we must assume he would want to look as attractive as possible. If the person usually dressed before breakfast, try to continue this routine. Introduce as little change as possible. Avoid delays or

70

interruptions in the morning routine, but allow lots of time to prevent rushing the person.

There are no recommended modes of dress. Whatever is easy, appropriate, and familiar is usually best. Some suggested strategies include:

- Create a feeling of privacy for the person.
- Encourage the person to participate in getting dressed. Simply handing the person his shirt may trigger an automatic cue to put it on.
- If the person is easily overwhelmed by many choices, offer only one or two choices in outfits. Clothing seldom worn can be removed from closets, reducing confusion.
- Keep the room as clear from clutter as possible, in order to lessen confusion.
- Label dresser drawers and closets, describing their contents.
- In the morning, lay out clothing in the order that they must be put on, making sure that all articles of clothing are right side out. This will help cue the person as to what to do first.
- If necessary, help to begin the activity by starting with an arm in one sleeve. This may be the only cue that is needed to finish putting on the shirt.
- Replace complicated buttons with velcro fasteners or zippers if fine motor co-ordination is becoming a problem. However, if a person has never used velcro before, it may create a problem rather than solve one.
- Use skirts or pants with an elastic waistband to facilitate ease of use, especially when needing to use the bathroom.
- Knee-high stockings or socks may be easier than nylons or pantyhose for women to manage, but

make sure they are not too tight on the top.

- Be sensitive to the person's reaction to mirrors or any reflective surfaces. Some people find the reflection in mirrors frightening, as they no longer recognize themselves or others.
- Periodically check the soles and heels of shoes and slippers for wear. Thin, worn soles can be slippery. Choose shoes and slippers that close easily.

Loss of Bladder/Bowel Control

Incontinence is the inability to control bladder and/or bowel elimination. This may occur during the middle to late stage, with bladder incontinence usually occurring earliest. It is important to consult your doctor, particularly if incontinence begins unusually early in the disease. Perhaps there is a medical problem such as a urine infection, which, when treated, can halt or decrease the problem of incontinence.

Keep a diary or chart
For several days write down the times accidents occur, the times the person successfully uses the toilet, and the times the person eat or drinks. Once you know when problems usually occur, you can set up a toileting schedule to prevent accidents.

Establish a regular bathroom routine
Set up a schedule for toileting and help the person stick to it. Remind the person or assist him to the bathroom every two hours, with special reminders when rising in the morning, after meals, and before bedtime. This is a sensitive issue, so be respectful when reminding the person. Encourage the person to drink lots of fluids

during the day, but reduce intake in the late evening.

Make sure the bathroom is easy to find

A clear sign, a picture of a toilet on the door, contrasting colours for fixtures, or a brightly painted door may help. Install a nightlight to guide the way at night. People who urinate in wastebaskets, closets, and flowerpots may be unable to locate the bathroom or remember the appropriate place. They are attracted to the container because of contrasting colour and accessibility.

Easy-to-remove clothing will help a person successfully complete toileting independently. Supplies available through drug stores, which may assist in coping with incontinence, include:

- Rubber sheets for the beds.
- Adult incontinence pads: if necessary, use of incontinence pads may only be needed at night and can be lessened at home during the day if the caregiver can prompt the person to use the washroom about once every two hours.
- Commode chair: good to have in the bedroom if the bathroom is not adjacent.
- Washable chair covers. If you fear a favourite chair or rug will be damaged, remove it.

Maintain dignity. Never attempt to shame the person into continence (bowel/bladder control). If it is necessary to use incontinence pads, never refer to them as diapers.

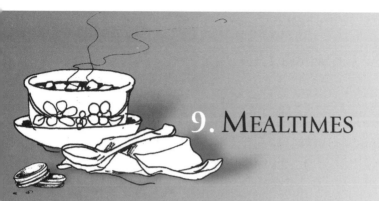

9. MEALTIMES

Both you and the person you are caring for need a balanced diet to avoid other illnesses and to cope with the stress of a chronic illness.

As with every activity, a regular routine is very important. Try to set meals for the same times during the day, and, if possible, involve the person in the preparation of the food. Stick to familiar and favourite foods. Every effort should be made to include the person in family meals. There is a special pleasure in eating with the family, and mealtimes can trigger many precious memories. Never comment on spilled food or in any way say anything that could cause embarrassment. Allow the person all the time necessary to finish eating, even if you must reheat the food. Just think how hard she is trying!

The Table and Utensils

- Ensure good posture to reduce the risk of choking.
- Add pepper and spices to food before serving, not at the table. Too many things on the table only add to the confusion.

- Serve small portions and only one course at a time. The person should only have one plate or bowl and a glass to deal with at a time.
- A damp cloth under the plate can prevent it from sliding. Using a bowl, instead of a plate, may decrease the potential for accidents and spills. Plates with raised rims are also good.
- If using a knife is difficult, cut up the meal beforehand into bite-size portions.
- Use plain-coloured plates, bowls, and placemats. Placemats should contrast in colour with any bowls or plates to help with perceptual problems.
- A barbecue apron or baker's apron will help with spills.
- Flexi-straws for liquids, and easy-grip handles for utensils, are available from drug stores, in the "Home Health Equipment" department.

Communication

- Use simple, one-step instructions, such as "pick up your fork," "put food on it." Demonstrating will help the person understand what you are saying.
- Eating your own meal with the person you are caring for provides visual cues for her, as well as reinforcing the social aspect of mealtimes.
- Use hand-on-hand guidance, if necessary, to initiate eating.
- Always tell the person what food you are giving her.

Agitation

- A very heavy chair at the table can make it difficult for someone who is restless to get up and down repeatedly.

 Mealtimes

- If agitated, stroke the person's shoulders and neck to help with relaxation. Try soft, relaxing music during the meal.
- Reduce noise and distractions in the dining area during meals.

Tips About Food

- Stick to familiar and favourite foods. These will help maintain interest.
- Avoid very hot foods. Use mugs or cups for soups.
- Put a date on food in the fridge and freezer.
- Select foods with sensory appeal—flavourful aromas, bright colour, and appealing textures.

There may be times when the person will reject food for no apparent reason. Do not argue or scold. Take the plate back to the kitchen, and then return with it in five minutes. By then, the person will probably have forgotten the unwillingness to eat and will consume the entire meal. If not, give essential fluids and wait until the next meal, or try a snack in between.

Caregivers should record any noticeable changes in the person's food and liquid intake, or food preferences. Always maintain a check on weight, making any necessary adjustments in diet should significant changes in weight occur.

As the Disease Progresses

As the disease progresses and difficulties arise, there is a loss of association between hunger pains and the need to eat. As co-ordination deteriorates, support independent eating as long as possible. Allow enough time. Adaptive, easy-grip utensils, dinnerware with food bumpers, and cups with spouts and plate grippers can help the person with worsening co-ordination. Provide finger foods such as cups of fruit, sandwiches, and cheese and crackers. They are easy to handle and nutritious. Resorting to finger foods is much better than taking over the task of feeding the person yourself. This can result in a tremendous loss of dignity for the person, and should be done only as a last resort.

The person may have difficulty swallowing and may need help with eating. Soft, familiar foods, such as eggs, casseroles, and soups, are a good choice. You may want to add nutritional drinks to ensure adequate nutrition. High-protein drinks increase calories as appetite decreases. Purée food in a blender to facilitate swallowing. Do not attempt to feed the person baby food directly from the jar. Serving from a bowl promotes dignity and respect. Do not hurry the eating process. It is a good time to show love and caring.

If the Person Requires Meal Assistance

- Make sure the person is seated in an upright position to avoid choking.
- Tell the person what food you are giving.
- Use deliberate, slow motions; never rush.
- Bring a spoonful of food within eye range and touch the person's mouth gently until it opens. If the person is restless, hold her right hand with your left to provide security.
- Remove the spoon from the person's mouth very slowly after each bite.
- Follow the person's cues indicating when she is ready for more.

• Liquids such as juice or milk can be more difficult to swallow than thick drinks, soups, or soft foods.

If and when the issue of tube-feeding has to be considered, take into account the ethical, religious, and emotional considerations of such an intervention. In many cases family consent is needed for a person who is unable to make her own decisions. In such cases an assessment must be made as to what the person would want for herself given the risks and benefits of the treatment. For people who are clearly and irreversibly deteriorating, and who are beyond a reasonable hope of recovery, it is ethically permissible not to begin this kind of feeding. Artificial eating carries risks that include aspiration, infection, fluid overload, removal of the tube by the person, and overall patient discomfort. There can be exceptions where tube-feeding may be beneficial. Talk to your physician about this.

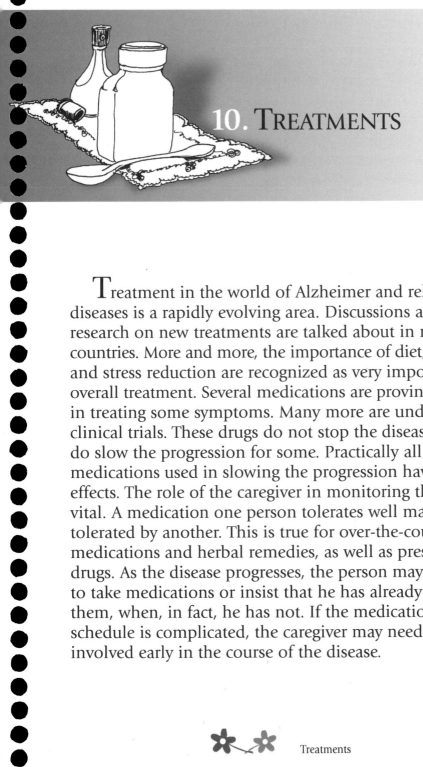

10. TREATMENTS

Treatment in the world of Alzheimer and related diseases is a rapidly evolving area. Discussions and research on new treatments are talked about in many countries. More and more, the importance of diet, exercise, and stress reduction are recognized as very important in overall treatment. Several medications are proving helpful in treating some symptoms. Many more are undergoing clinical trials. These drugs do not stop the disease, but do slow the progression for some. Practically all medications used in slowing the progression have side effects. The role of the caregiver in monitoring this is vital. A medication one person tolerates well may not be tolerated by another. This is true for over-the-counter medications and herbal remedies, as well as prescription drugs. As the disease progresses, the person may forget to take medications or insist that he has already taken them, when, in fact, he has not. If the medication schedule is complicated, the caregiver may need to be involved early in the course of the disease.

Aricept, Exelon, Reminyl

For people who are in the early to middle progression of the disease, the two first medications that became available in Canada were Aricept and Exelon. This was followed a couple of years later by Reminyl. Ask your physician or call the Alzheimer Society to get an update of what is currently available. Donepezil (with the trade name of Aricept) and Rivastigmine (with the trade name of Exelon) have been approved by Health Canada to help in the treatment of Alzheimer Disease. These drugs are not a cure for Alzheimer Disease, as they do not affect the underlying degenerative process of the disease. Many more drugs will likely be approved over the next few years. Another that was approved in Canada in 2003 was Galantamine (with the trade name of Reminyl).

The drugs that have been approved for the treatment of symptoms in people with mild to moderate Alzheimer Disease are drugs that have been classified as "cholinesterase inhibitors." In the brains of people with Alzheimer and related diseases there is a progressive degeneration of nerve cells. Particularly notable is a degeneration of cells that make acetylcholine, a chemical thought to be important for learning and memory. People with this disease also have lower brain levels of acetylcholine. The new class of drugs acts by decreasing the activity of acetylcholinesterase, an enzyme whose function is to break down acetylcholine. It is believed that because the medications reduce the breakdown of acetylcholine, it will lead to an increase in the level of this chemical in the brain. The potential beneficial effect could lessen as the disease progresses and when fewer cells are available to make acetylcholine.

Possible Side Effects

Along with their beneficial effect, these treatments may cause some undesirable reactions. The most common side effects include nausea, diarrhea, insomnia, vomiting, muscle cramps, fatigue, and loss of appetite. In clinical studies these effects were often mild, and generally went away with continued treatment.

Suggestions to Assist in Supervision of Treatments or Medications

- Contact the doctor immediately if you notice any symptoms that you do not understand, or find distressing.
- Consult the doctor and attempt to keep the routine as simple as possible.
- Use daily or weekly dispenser cases. If the daily medications are prepared for the person in advance and placed in such containers, he may be able to manage medications independently in the early stages.
- Present medications to the person in a positive manner, avoiding the impression of giving orders:
  "It is time to take your pills now. Dr. Jones wants you to have them so you will feel well."
- If pills are resisted, check with the doctor to see if the medication is available in liquid form or if it can be crushed and mixed with ice cream or applesauce. It is important to check before crushing pills, as the effect of some medications is drastically changed with crushing.
- If the person lives alone, make and maintain a list of medications. Prepare daily pill dosages in special

containers. Prepare dated or colour-coded "tapes" (masking tape over the pills) for each dose. Check frequently to be sure they are being taken properly. Phone call reminders may be a good idea. Throw out any unused or outdated medications. Talk to a Home Care Nurse.

- Monitor alcohol use. Check with the doctor about the interaction of alcohol with prescribed drugs. For people with this disease, the interaction of alcohol with particular drugs may be especially pronounced.
- The pharmacist is a professional who can provide information about medications, especially their interactions with each other and with over-the-counter products and alcohol. The pharmacist is usually easier to access, and sees his role as providing this type of public information.
- Keep a record of drugs that have caused allergic or other reactions in the past. For some people, medications have an opposite effect and can cause increased agitation.
- Keep the phone number of the Poison Control Centre close to your phone.

In addition to being sure that medications are being taken as directed, the caregiver has another important role: monitoring the potential side effects of newly prescribed medications and the interaction of various drugs with each other or with over-the-counter drugs. Since the person may have a reduced ability to communicate verbally, the caregiver must be attuned to any changes in behaviour, such as drowsiness, drooling, incontinence, or increased agitation. This is a very complicated issue that should be discussed with the doctor or nurse and/or pharmacist.

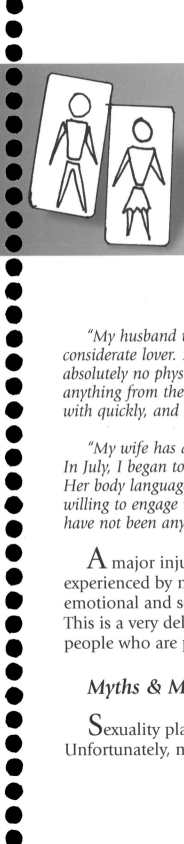

11. SEXUALITY

"My husband was a wonderful, tender, thoughtful, and considerate lover. For two years, since he became ill, I've had absolutely no physical or emotional satisfaction. I don't get anything from the sexual experience. We do it and get it over with quickly, and that's that!"

"My wife has always been affectionate to the nth degree. In July, I began to notice a change in her attitude about sex. Her body language suggested that she was not interested or willing to engage in sexual activity. Since November 21, there have not been any intimate relations."

A major injustice of Alzheimer and related diseases experienced by married couples is the increasing loss of emotional and sexual intimacy as the disease progresses. This is a very delicate and sensitive subject for many people who are personally experiencing these losses.

Myths & Misconceptions

Sexuality plays a vital part in all of our lives. Unfortunately, myths and misinformation can negatively affect sexual beliefs and behaviour, often with devastating consequences. For example, some older people accept the notion that one's sex life should end after a certain age, especially if they have a disease like Alzheimer Disease, and they are reluctant to seek information or treatment for a sexual problem. Often, older people are not told about normal changes with age; or the impact that a loss of privacy, medications, or medical conditions can have on sexual desire or performance; or the significance of emotional factors such as lowered self-esteem, depression, or anxiety. This information alone can be therapeutic, and the knowledge can enhance sexual functioning and emotional well-being.

The onset of sexual problems may not result solely from the progression of dementia. Sexual problems may be early warning signs of other health concerns left unattended, like anemia, alcoholism, diabetes, or even constipation. One caregiver reported that unrelieved constipation caused painful intercourse for his wife. When treated, she was able to resume relations with the same degree of pleasure previously experienced.

Common myths and misconceptions include:

- *Prostate surgery, heart problems, and other conditions mean the end of an active sex life.* Many misconceptions about prostate disease, heart problems, and other conditions lead to unnecessary fears, and decisions to cease sexual activity. Men are sometimes reluctant to consent to prostate surgery because of the mistaken notion that it inevitably leads to impotence. Although this happens in some cases, recent research and medical techniques are reassuring. See a specialist for specific answers to your questions. Couples are sometimes hesitant about resuming sexual relations after one partner has had a heart attack, for fear of causing another. A doctor or nurse should discuss this as part of a discharge plan.

- *Many older people are not interested in sex, especially after a diagnosis of dementia.* People who have had an active sexual life often will continue to need affection and sexual expression after diagnosis of Alzheimer Disease. Depending on the personalities of the couple involved, the sexual relationship will not necessarily change until the disease progresses further.

- *Orgasm is the primary purpose of sexual activity.* Couples report that the warmth and intimacy from sharing are critical ingredients in a relationship. Touching, tenderness, cuddling, appreciating, and attending to each other's sensuality needs can be the essence of a good relationship, and may be more important than orgasm.

- *Alcohol increases sexual performance.* Alcohol appears to be helpful because it relaxes the person and causes less inhibition. However, it is a depressant and actually interferes with sexual performance. Also, use of alcohol in combination with other medications can result in various other reactions or side-effects.

- *Older people, and particularly persons who have been married for many years and have enjoyed an active sex life, do not need sex education or information.* We live in a time when the media seems saturated with sex, in a time where rules governing behaviour are extremely vague, and in a society that tolerates different lifestyles to a greater degree than ever before. This all suggests a more sexually knowledgeable public. Surprisingly, this is not the case. Research and clinical evidence suggest that all age groups, including older people, are often lacking in even basic sex information. Many older people grew up in a time when sex education was unavailable. Some lack vital information about the changes that accompany certain illnesses, surgical procedures, and the aging process itself. Many questions or concerns that people have could be cleared up with accurate information, resulting in very positive consequences. Talk to your doctor or contact the Alzheimer Society for information or referral.

- *Inappropriate and excessive sexual behaviour is a common symptom of Alzheimer Disease.* It is, in fact, rare. In most instances the problem is not a case of inappropriate sexual behaviour, but a case of not understanding the environment or the actions of others. For example, a person advanced in the disease may undress in a public place because she is unaware of being in a public place.

Sexual Functioning

Loving and being loved in return are basic human needs. People affected by this disease may feel an increased need for the reassurance and comfort that comes from being held, touched, and loved, and from receiving the loving attention of another person. Sexuality can be broadly defined to include comfort, security, touch, and sharing, as well as the physical aspects of sexual activity. Many couples find a fulfilling sexual relationship that does not include sexual intercourse. The nature of the relationship is not important, as long as it is mutually satisfying to both parties. What is important is when there is a change that becomes problematic for one or both partners.

Sexual problems related to this disease are varied and complex. Some couples report that the bond between them is strengthened because of the challenges of the disease. They become more devoted to each other in their commitment to face increasing losses in their familiar relationship, while taking on new roles and adjusting to a relationship that is now being shaped by a disease over which they have little control. As the person becomes less able to play a familiar role, the spouse learns to adapt, using various techniques, aids, or attitudes to nurture and maintain the relationship in a mutually satisfying way. Other people report sexual problems of varying kinds. Most problems are troublesome to the degree that they occur at inappropriate times or with an inappropriate person. Behaviours are sometimes construed to be sexual when in fact they may be prompted by other motives.

The caregiving spouse may report concerns in one or more of the following areas:

- The person may express an interest in sexual activity, but may do so in a selfish or unacceptable manner. No caregiver should suffer physical, emotional, or verbal abuse. Talk to your physician if this is happening. There are no magic cures for this behaviour, but there are techniques to lessen the impact of such behaviour. Other people may become frightened or threatened when they no longer recognize the caregiving spouse.
- The caregiver may become dismayed or embarrassed about the sexual relationship because of drastic changes in the partner's personality, hygiene, interactions with others, or new sexual behaviours.

- The caregiver may be too exhausted or depressed from the physical demands of caregiving, so that even when the person is willing and capable of participating in a familiar way, the caregiver is not interested and may feel guilty about not being emotionally available.
- The caregiver is often expected to be caring and nurturing. It may be difficult to be loving and affectionate under such trying circumstances, particularly when the person has become not only "different but difficult." Caregivers may feel alone in their concerns and questions. Physicians may neglect to ask about such concerns, or dismiss them as not being very important when compared with the seriousness of the disease. Caregivers must make it clear that this is an important issue. If your physician is not sympathetic to your problem, your Alzheimer Society can help. Counsellors are available to help you sort out your feelings and to help you find alternatives to problems you are facing.
- Alzheimer and related diseases can affect sexual functioning in many ways. The response of sexual partners to these effects depends on the progression of the disease, the strength and length of the relationship, the importance that intercourse has held in life-long expressions of sexual intimacy, and many personality and social factors. Alzheimer Disease frequently causes a reduction in sexual arousal and the ability to maintain arousal for both men and women. These problems may be solved medically and a doctor should be consulted.
- A classic symptom of Alzheimer Disease is the loss of initiative. This loss of initiative has a profound effect on expressing affection, including sexual

intimacy. In the earlier progression of the disease, the affected partner may continue to be able to engage in sexual relations if the well partner initiates the lovemaking. For some who are unfamiliar with this role, this may be uncomfortable. Discussion with a sensitive and caring health professional may be helpful.

- Some couples can develop ways of communicating affection based upon years of common living that transcend the impairments of the disease. Examples include visiting, going for walks, listening to music, and sharing a special meal. These familiar events may help trigger expressions of affection. In general, maintaining traditional times together, continuing the ways in which togetherness and affection have always been expressed, even if they must be done in slightly different ways, can initiate expressions of affection.

Sexuality is a sensitive and difficult topic for some. It is important to discuss your feelings with friends, relatives, or health professionals. The Alzheimer Society can help.

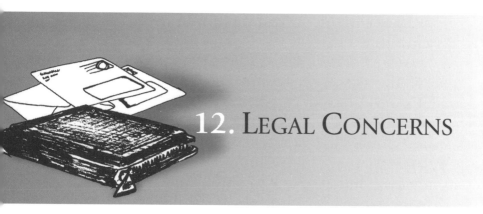

12. LEGAL CONCERNS

It is essential to put legal and financial affairs in order immediately upon hearing of a diagnosis of Alzheimer or a related disease.

When a person is diagnosed, it is essential to move quickly to ensure that the financial affairs can be looked after as the disease progresses. To wait until the disease progresses is to risk having a bank or other institution assert that the person is incompetent to make financial decisions. At that point, only the courts can declare incompetence and for legal and financial purposes appoint another person or persons to look after the financial affairs.

During the early progression of the disease, the person should participate in legal and financial planning, since it is still his right and privilege to do so. The family may not be aware of the location of some legal documents or may not know of all legal transactions that have taken place. If discussed early enough, there will be no surprises for anyone. If you must take over the legal and financial matters of someone who has Alzheimer Disease, it will be easier if you know the person's wishes beforehand.

This will also help ease any sense of guilt you may be experiencing, now or in the future. Do not put off visiting a lawyer to seek legal advice on issues such as Wills and Power of Attorney. A lawyer can explain the importance of Health Care Directives and update you on what is happening in your province or state around consent to treatment.

Wills/Living Wills

A Will is a legal document that states how a person wants his assets divided after death. It assures the person's wishes are carried out. A person with Alzheimer or a related disease must make a Will before he becomes too ill and is unable to make sound decisions. The caregiver should also have an updated Will. If you have left your entire, or partial, estate to the person diagnosed, or if you have named that person as your Executor, he will not be able to handle these responsibilities in the future. Talk to your lawyer about changes you may want to make. You may want to set up a trust in your Will for the person with the disease, in case you predecease him. Make sure your family knows where your Will is located.

Like Power of Attorney, a Living Will is another way of assuring that a person's wishes are carried out during his lifetime, should he become incapacitated. It can give general directions or specific wishes about medical procedures that he may or may not want. A Living Will may also express a wish that family members not participate in decisions relating to medical treatment. Family members will be relieved to know that decisions were made when the person was of sound mind. A Will, Power of Attorney, and Living Will can be prepared on very short notice. They do not even require a visit to a lawyer's office and are among the few services for which some lawyers may make a house call.

Power of Attorney

This is a legal document allowing you to give another person the authority to act on your behalf. This still allows you control of your affairs, and you can still act on your own behalf as well. When granting a Power of Attorney, you must be competent and fully understand the agreement at the time it is written.

A Power of Attorney can be simple or enduring:
- Simple: This type of document lasts as long as the person setting it up remains able to understand and agree to the arrangement. A simple Power of Attorney ends when the person becomes incompetent.
- Enduring: A person may assign to someone else the power to continue making decisions even after the grantor has become incompetent. If the enduring Power of Attorney is authorized early enough in the illness, it should be sufficient to protect and manage the estate until after death.

The person holding Power of Attorney must be at least 19 years of age. A Power of Attorney can be general or specific. A general Power of Attorney gives the person authority to act on behalf of another person in all legal and financial matters, such as signing cheques or selling the house. A specific Power of Attorney gives the attorney power to carry out specific acts only, such as power to deal with a bank account. It is an important document giving a lot of power to someone else, so it is important that the authority be given to someone you know and trust.

It is recommended that the Power of Attorney be prepared and witnessed by a lawyer, thus providing added security should the Power of Attorney ever be challenged in court. You may want to consider naming an Alternate Attorney, as a back-up, should the person with the Power of Attorney be unable to carry on the task. Banks and other financial institutions usually have their own Power of Attorney forms. If you are buying or selling land under a Power of Attorney, you must register the Power at the Registry of Deeds.

Establishment of a Trust

Among the options available is the establishment of a trust. In order to establish the trust, the person must be deemed sufficiently competent by the lawyer to make the decision because it has enduring significance. By establishing the trust, the person transfers legal ownership of the listed assets to the trust and the trustees named in it. Because the assets are legally transferred, the trustees have complete responsibility and discretion in the administration of the assets. It is incumbent then upon the trustees to look after the assets for the person for whom the trust has been established. This permits the trustees to pay all bills and administer investments on behalf of the trust. While the trustees are the legal owners of all the assets in the trust, there are no tax implications for them as the assets still are deemed to be the income of the person in whose name the trust is established.

General Points to Consider
- Credit cards held in the name of a person with Alzheimer Disease should be cancelled and destroyed to avoid irrational purchases, loss, or theft.
- Ownership of an automobile should not be with the person with Alzheimer or a related illness. It may affect the status of the insurance on the vehicle.

- A joint bank account that requires only one signature will allow the caregiver to withdraw money as needed.
- It is possible to apply to Health Canada to have Old Age Security and Canada Pension cheques paid to the caregiver in trust for the person.

For more information, contact your family lawyer or your local community legal information association.

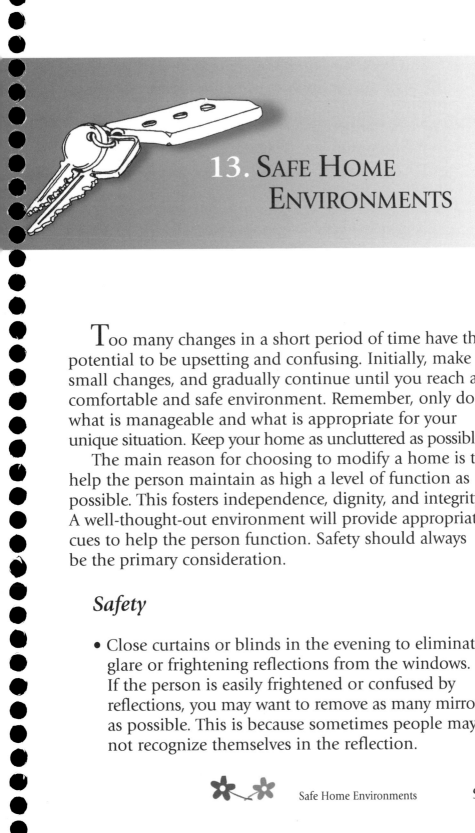

13. SAFE HOME ENVIRONMENTS

Too many changes in a short period of time have the potential to be upsetting and confusing. Initially, make small changes, and gradually continue until you reach a comfortable and safe environment. Remember, only do what is manageable and what is appropriate for your unique situation. Keep your home as uncluttered as possible.

The main reason for choosing to modify a home is to help the person maintain as high a level of function as possible. This fosters independence, dignity, and integrity. A well-thought-out environment will provide appropriate cues to help the person function. Safety should always be the primary consideration.

Safety

* Close curtains or blinds in the evening to eliminate glare or frightening reflections from the windows. If the person is easily frightened or confused by reflections, you may want to remove as many mirrors as possible. This is because sometimes people may not recognize themselves in the reflection.

- Slide a bolt from the closet door into the floor if rummaging may present hazards. Provide a rummaging box.
- Provide a secure area for medications.
- Install handrails on stairways and in bathrooms.
- Install extra locks on exit doors and windows in places where they are not easily noticed.
- Ensure continued update with the *Safely Home— Alzheimer Wandering Registry*.
- Remove dangerous objects or substances, especially from under the kitchen sink, and in the bathroom cabinet.
- Adjust appliances with the potential to cause burns or fire (for example, removing fuses from stove, lowering hot water temperature, putting a lock on the thermostat).
- Add a fence to the backyard and a safety lock to the gate.
- Remove sharp-cornered furniture and sharp objects.
- Eliminate scatter mats.
- Keep outside lights off at night to discourage interest in going outside.
- Mark windows and glass doors with stickers or hanging ornaments to help with easier visibility.
- Put plastic plugs in all unused electrical outlets.
- If the person smokes, try to provide supervision and add a little water in all the ashtrays.
- Put away power tools, scissors, and any other items that can no longer be safely used without supervision.
- Give away poisonous houseplants that might be eaten.
- Do not wax floors; the slippery finish is more treacherous and the shininess may be confusing.
- Install rubber treads on uncarpeted stairs to improve traction.

- Mark the edge of steps with contrasting colours.
- Add a safety railing on outside steps or along the veranda.
- Install bells or an electronic alarm system on exit doors.
- Remove visible inside locks from doors to eliminate the possibility of the person locking herself inside.
- Place labels (words or pictures) on cupboard, closet, and bathroom doors to encourage independence.

Furniture/Furnishings

- Hang pictures that the person enjoys low enough to be appreciated.
- Provide a comfortable chair near a favourite window and close to quiet activity so the person can feel included
- Make furniture as stationary and stable as possible by fixing any wobbly legs or arms on chairs.
- Move the furniture away from the middle of rooms, making space for the person to pace or walk.
- Use chairs with arms. If purchasing new pieces of furniture, make sure they have rounded corners.
- Decrease general clutter, removing any unnecessary obstacles so it is easier to get around.

Bathroom

- Consider a chair for inside the tub or shower to help with balance.
- Slide-proof the bottom of the tub or use a coloured rubber mat.
- Install a grab bar by both the toilet and the tub

 Safe Home Environments

(or clamp a grip handle to the side of the tub).

- Keep shampoo and other potentially harmful liquids out of the bathroom in case they are swallowed; bring them in only when needed.
- Use contrasting coloured tape around the edge of the tub to help define its edges and depth.
- Install washable, rubber-backed bathroom carpeting to reduce chances of slipping on a wet bathroom floor.
- Consider installing a raised toilet seat, if helpful.
- Use contrasting colours in the bathroom so fixtures will stand out from the wall colour.
- Use a deep soap container so that the soap will not fall into the tub or onto the floor.
- Always leave a nightlight turned on in the bathroom.

Kitchen

- Adjust the kitchen stove, so it cannot be used without supervision, by removing knobs and fuses, or have an electrician install a safety switch that is out of sight.
- Remove sharp knives, electric kettle, and other small appliances (this does not have to be elaborate— simply put the items out of sight).
- Get an electric, whistling kettle that has an automatic shut-off.
- Have all cleaning products and detergents locked up and out of reach.
- Use safety latches on cupboard doors if necessary.
- Remove the rug from under the table where you eat. It may be too difficult for the person to push a chair back and this may cause a bad fall. It is also easier to clean up a bare floor.
- Remove items that are precious and breakable, such as ornaments and delicate antiques.

Bedroom

- Remove the bed frame, so that a fall out of bed will not be so damaging.
- Relocate bedrooms to the main floor, if necessary, as early in the disease as possible. As the disease progresses, changes in routine can sometimes cause problems even when you are trying to prevent them. If possible, try to locate the bedroom close to a bathroom.
- Use nightlights in the bedroom, and leading to the bathroom. Putting lights in these two areas of the house, while leaving the rest of the house dark at night, may prevent the person from wandering away from the security of the lighted areas.

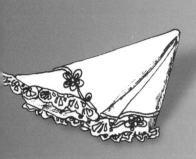

14. LATE PROGRESSION OF ALZHEIMER DISEASE

As caregivers watch the decline in abilities of the person being cared for, they experience intense emotions, pain, helplessness, and confusion. Making decisions is hard but necessary. When coping with a long-term and progressive illness, it is important to consider options for the future well ahead of time. Some caregivers choose to care at home until the end, while others know they need to make the decision to continue to care with outside help. This can be with assistance at home or choosing a facility where staff have special training. Talk to your Alzheimer Society about the differences between private and government/public care facilities. Often there is a different admission process for each. Request a copy of the *Guidelines for Care* from the Alzheimer Society. During the early stage of this disease, the person may be able to indicate any preferences for future care, making potentially painful decisions much easier for you. It takes time to secure admission to a nursing care facility, and planning ahead is important. Pre-planning will help you avoid a potential crisis situation, if you come to a point where you can no longer provide adequate care and you need the service of a care facility.

Death and Dying

By the time people enter the later stages of this disease, their caregivers are often nearing exhaustion. Whether caring at home, or visiting your family member in a nursing home or hospital, ongoing care issues are still a priority.

- Physical touch is a very important means of communication. Holding hands, gentle massage, using textures, and continuing to talk about family events communicate love and caring. (Look for responses from the person in such areas as facial expression and body posture.)
- Play treasured music from years past. Read favourite passages, poems, and stories.
- Maintain normal range of movement by getting the person up and out of bed as frequently as possible. Short walks, little visits, and laughter will all provide some level of stimulation and comfort. Without movement, and change of position, painful contractures develop in the arms, hands, and legs; breathing and heart function deteriorate, and the skin breaks down.
- Consider hiring full-time help, if affordable. Talk to the Alzheimer Society about other options for getting support.
- If caring at home, request regular help from community resources, such as Meals on Wheels, and accept offers of assistance from other family members and friends. Obtain a list of services from the Alzheimer Society.
- Avoid becoming too isolated in caregiving. Now is a time when you will need friends and family around you.

- Inquire about palliative care options.
- Talk to your physician or the Alzheimer Society about the Brain Bank Donation program.
- Consider whether autopsy will be a choice. This decision should not be left to the emotional time surrounding death. Talk to your doctor.
  "At the time we didn't understand the need for research. Now we wish we'd had the autopsy done."
- Discuss resuscitation measures with staff. Many people are very clear about their desire not to have "heroic measures."
- Stay in tune with your feelings and be involved in a support group and/or counselling.

The Grieving Process

Accepting death as a part of life is something we will all have to face. Grieving is painful and involves our entire being. With this disease, both the caregiver and the person receiving care experience the effects of losses daily. Grieving involves the reactions and responses to loss, and is necessary and healthy. It is about letting go and saying good-bye. Healing is a process that takes time. It is hard work, but allows an integration of life lessons that stretch your body and soul to new awareness.

The grieving process is unique to each person, but will conjure up many similar feelings and symptoms. Guilt, depression, sadness, bitterness, anger, doubtfulness, restlessness, anxiousness, loneliness, and apathy are among the painful feelings. Crying, sleepless nights, weight loss, knots in the stomach, headaches, and other physical ailments are not uncommon. Because this disease can last such a long time, there can be frequent episodes of grieving. It has been described as "the funeral that never ends." Sometimes people feel like they are on a roller coaster. During the process of grieving:

- Seek and accept help early in the process.
- Allow and accept all feelings. Naming and normalizing feelings can reduce fear and give a sense of control.
- Talk to a trusted person about the feelings; nurture friendships.
- Consider individual counselling, spiritual direction, and/or a peer support system.
- Obtain recommended readings.
- Keep a diary or journal.
- Consider personal development courses or others that may be of interest.
- Explore the strength of forgiveness—the healing of gently forgiving yourself when you are burdened with unrealistic expectations, or when you feel angry because of the challenges you face as a caregiver.
- Be kind to yourself. Do something special. Set a goal.
- Consider helping another who has just started on the path you are finishing.
- Set new goals.
- If feeling stuck, call your Alzheimer Society for support, suggestions, or referral.

How you have dealt with previous losses will directly affect how you grieve the dying of your family member. If grieving was put on the back burner in the past, it is time to allow yourself new ways of grieving that will enable you to deal with reality while still maintaining energy to care.

"…And we ourselves shall be loved for a while and forgotten. But the love will have been enough; all those impulses of love return to the love that made them. Even memory is not necessary for love. There is a land of the living and a land of the dead, and the bridge is love, the only survival, the only meaning."

—Thornton Wilder

15. PROVINCIAL ALZHEIMER SOCIETIES IN CANADA

Alzheimer Society of Prince Edward Island
166 Fitzroy Street, Charlottetown, PE C1A 7K4
Tel: (902) 628-2257 Fax: (902) 368-2715
E-mail: society@alzpei.ca

Alzheimer Society of Newfoundland and Labrador, Inc.
687 Water Street - PO Box 37013, St. John's, NF A1E 1C2
Tel: (709) 576-0608 Fax: (709) 576-0798
E-mail: sharing@avalon.nf.ca

Alzheimer Society of Nova Scotia
5954 Spring Garden Road, Halifax, NS B3H 1Y7
Tel: (902) 422-7961 Fax: (902) 422-7971
E-mail: alzheimer@ns.sympatico.ca

Alzheimer Society of New Brunswick
PO Box 1553, Station A, Fredericton, NB E3B 5G2
Tel: (506) 459-4280 Tel: Info and Referral (800) 664-8411
Fax: (506) 452-0313
E-mail: info@alzheimernb.ca

Federation of Quebec Alzheimer Societies
5165, rue Sherbrooke ouest, bur. 200 Montreal, QC H4A 1T6
Tel: (514) 369-7891 (888) MEMOIRE (636-6473)
Fax: (514) 369-7900
E-mail: info_fqsa@alzheimerquebec.ca

Alzheimer Society of Ontario
1200 Bay St., Suite 202, Toronto, ON M5R 2A5
Tel: (416) 967-5900 Fax: (416) 967-3826
E-mail: alzheimeront@sympatico.ca

Alzheimer Society of Manitoba
120 Donald St., Unit 10, Winnipeg, MB R3C 4G2
Tel: (204) 943-6622 Fax: (204) 942-5408
E-mail: alzmb@alzheimer.mb.ca

Alzheimer Society of Saskatchewan
2550 - 12th Ave., Suite 301, Regina, SK S4P 3X1
Tel: (306) 949-4141 (800) 263-3367 Fax: (306) 949-3069
E-mail: info@alzheimer.sk.ca

Alzheimer Society of Alberta
2323 - 32 Ave. N.E., Suite 220, Calgary, AB T2E 6Z3
Tel: (403) 250-1303 Fax: (403) 250-8241
E-mail: province@alzheimer.ab.ca

Alzheimer Society of British Columbia
#300 - 828 West 8th Avenue., Vancouver, BC V5Z 1E2
Tel: (604) 681-6530 Fax: (604) 669-6907
E-mail: info@alzheimerbc.org

Alzheimer Society of Canada
20 Eglinton Ave. West, Suite 1200, Toronto, Ontario M4R 1K8
Tel: (416) 488-8772 Fax: (416) 488-3778
National Web Site: www.alzheimer.ca

16. ALZHEIMER ASSOCIATIONS AROUND THE WORLD

Country	Telephone Number	E-mail Address
Argentina	+54 11 4671 1187	alma@satlink.com.ar
Australia	+61 2 6254 4233	glenn@alzheimers.org.au
Austria	+43 1 332 5166	alzheimeraustria@via.at
Belgium	+32 4 225 8793	henry.sabine@skynet.be
Brazil	+55 11 270 8791	abraz@abraz.com.br
Canada	+1 416 488 8772	info@alzheimer.ca
China	+8610 6521 2012	xuxh@public.bta.net.cn
Chile	+56 2 236 0846	alzchile@mi.terra.cl
Colombia	+57 1 348 199	alzheimercolombia@hotmail.com
Costa Rica	+506 290 28 44	ascada@msn.com
Cuba	+537 220974	inmo@teleda.get.tur.cu
Cyprus	+357 4 627 104	alzhcyprus@yahoo.com
Czech Republic	+420 2 88 36 76	Petr.Veleta@gerontocentrum.cz
Denmark	+45 39 40 04 88	post@alzheimer.dk
Dominican Republic	+1 809 544 1711	dr.pedro@codetel.net.do
Ecuador	+593 2 2594 997	gustavomatute@andinanet.net
Egypt	+202 392 0074	amashour2002@yahoo.com
El Salvador	+503 237 0787	ricardolopez@vianet.com.sv
Finland	+358 9 6226 200	tarja.tapaninen@alzheimer.fi
France	+33 1 42 97 52 41	contact@francealzheimer.com
Germany	+49 30315 057 33	deutsche.alzheimer.ges@t-online.de
Greece	+30 31 925802	alzhass@med.auth.gr
Guatemala	+502 2 381122	alzguate@quetzal.net
Hong Kong SAR	+852 27943010	info@hkada.org.hk
Iceland	+354 533 1088	faas@alzheimer.is
India	+91 488 523801	alzheimer@md2.vsnl.net.in
Indonesia	+62 21 8730179	nasrun@indosat.net.id
Ireland	+353 1 284 6616	info@alzheimer.ie
Israel	+972 3 578 7660	misrad@alz-il.net

Italy	+39 02 809767	alzit@tin.it
Japan	+81 75 811 8195	office@alzheimer.or.jp
Korea	+82 2 431 9963	afcde01@unitel.co.kr
Luxembourg	+352 421 676	info@alzheimer.lu
Malaysia	+603 2260 3158	alzheimers@pd.jaring.my
Mexico	+771 71 9 47 52	fedma2002@hotmail.com
Netherlands	+31 30 659 6900	info@alzheimer-ned.nl
New Zealand	+64 3 365 1590	nationaloffice@alzheimers.org.nz
Nigeria	+234 46 463663	tifine@infoweb.abs.net
Norway	+47 23 12 00 00	post@nasjonalforeningen.no
Pakistan	+92 42 759 6589	info@alz.org.pk
Panama		hopemil@sinfo.net
Peru	+511 448 2237	magasc@terra.com.pe
Philippines	+632 723 1039	adap@alzphilippines.com
Poland	+48 22 622 11 22	alzheimer_pl@hotmail.com
Portugal	+351 21 361 0460	alzheimer@oninet.pt
Puerto Rico	+1 787 727 4151	alzheimerpr@alzheimerpr.org
Romania	+402 1 686 3470	contact@alz.ro
Russia	+7 095 324 9615	gavrilova@dionis.iasnet.ru
Scotland	+44 131 243 1453	alzheimer@alzscot.org
Singapore	+65 353 8734	alzheimers.tp@pacific.net.sg
Slovak Republic	+421 7 594 13353	nilunova@savba.sk
South Africa	+27 11 478 2234	alzheimerssa@icon.co.za
Spain	+34 948 1745 17	alzheimer@cin.es
Sri Lanka	+94 1 583488	alzheimers_foundation@serendib.ws
Sweden	+46 46 14 73 18	info@alzheimerforeningen.nu
Switzerland	+41 24 426 2000	alz@bluewin.ch
Thailand	+66 2 880 8542	
Trinidad & Tobago	+1 868 622 6134	klbtt@yahoo.com
Turkey	+90 212 224 41 89	muratemre@superonline.com
Uganda	+256 486 22290	adasuga@talk21.com
Ukraine	+380 44 431 0526	bachinskaya@geront.kiev.ua
United Kingdom	+44 20 7306 0606	enquires@alzheimers.org.uk
United States	+1 312 335 8700	info@alz.org
Uruguay	+5982 400 8797	audasur@adinet.com.uy
Venezuela	+58 212 4146129	alzven@cantv.net
Yugoslavia	+381 11 361 4122	dpavlovic@drenik.net
Zimbabwe	+263 4 703 423	suecox@ecoweb.co.zw

Every attempt has been made to verify the accuracy of this information at the time of publication. It will be updated as the book is reprinted.

ACKNOWLEDGEMENTS

I gratefully acknowledge the following people who reviewed the manuscript, many of whom provided suggestions that have been incorporated into this *Guide*.

Laurie Brinklow, The Acorn Press

Prince Edward Island Reviewers

Lorraine Begley	Doug Cameron	Dr. Bernice Bell
Dr. Tom Connor	Clive Cudmore	Dr. Doug Cudmore
Janet Doiron	Janet Keough	Eric Kipping
Lloyd Lockerby	Clara MacLeod	Henry MacWilliams
Pat Malone	Dr. Reg Hutchings	Maureen Paquet
Gerard Murnaghan	Florence Rossiter	Bonnie Sherren
Margie Stewart	Marilyn Sutherland	Dr. Lamont Sweet
Jill Sweet	Marcianne Gamauf	Arnold Winsor
Dr. Howard Zacharias	Dianne Winsor	Dr. Alfred Morais

Canadian Reviewers

Dr. Lise Hébért	—Quebec
Gloria McIlveen	—New Brunswick
Joan McKell	—New Brunswick
Gerard Murphy & Janet Johnston	—Nova Scotia
Anne Hallisey & Donna Dill	—Nova Scotia
Shirley Lucas	—Newfoundland
Peggy Viel	—Alberta
Dr. Jo Ann Miller	—British Columbia
Joanne Michael & Carol Dyck	—Saskatchewan
Wendy Schettler	—Manitoba
Shelley Vaillancourt	—Ontario
Ilona Horgan & Barbara Snelgrove	—Alzheimer Society of Canada

INDEX

A

abuse 87
alcohol 16, 82, 84, 85
Alzheimer Disease
      definition 24–7
      diagnosis 14, 16, 17
      duration 25, 28
      early detection 14, 17, 18
      progression 28–31, 79
      symptoms 14–6, 24, 25, 26
      testing for 14, 15
      treatments 79–82
agnosia 31
anxiety 58
apraxia 31
Aricept 80
autopsy 14, 102

B

bathing 65–9, 97–8
bathroom, using. *See* washroom, using
behaviour, change in 10, 14, 26, 29, 39, 50–64, 76–7, 100
bladder/bowel control 31, 72–3, 82
Brain Bank Donation Program 102
brain, damage to 24–27, 80

C

caffeine 58, 59
care facilities 20, 44, 100, 102
care for caregivers 18–23, 47–8, 59, 88, 100, 101
clothing 30, 53, 56, 60, 70–2, 73
College of Physicians and Surgeons 48–9

communication
        importance of 17, 20, 30, 33, 39–49, 51, 75
        non-verbal 40, 42, 43–4, 54, 77, 82, 101
confusion 12, 29–31, 40, 45, 50, 51, 52, 55
conversation, tips for 39–44, 47
counselling 27, 45, 88, 103

D

death and dying 31, 100–3
defensive behaviour 50–5
dementia, definition of 24
denial 17
dental care 69–70
depression 26, 30, 51, 59, 88
diagnostic imaging 14
diaries 14, 72, 103
dignity 10, 19, 28, 32, 43, 65, 68, 95
distraction 54, 61, 63, 68
dressing 65, 70–2
driving 12, 30, 55–6
drug reactions 15, 16

E

emergencies 53, 54, 82
environment
        adapting 9, 10, 26, 95–9
        changes to 61, 62
Ethical Guidelines for Communicating the Diagnosis 17
Exelon 80
exercise 37, 38, 52, 57, 58, 60, 61, 63, 79, 101

F

family, role of 12, 14, 16–23, 26, 29, 45, 55, 74
financial considerations 17, 20, 94–4
food 31, 38, 54, 58, 59, 63, 74–8
footware 72
furniture 96, 97

G

games 38
gardening 37
grief counselling 19, 102–3
grieving 102–3
Guidelines for Care 100
guilt, feelings of 17, 20

H

hobbies 37, 38
Home Care 69, 101
hospitalization 44–9
household chores 38
humour, importance of 21, 28, 34, 40

I

incontinence. *See* bladder/bowel control
independence, importance of 13, 19, 20, 65, 95
intimacy 43, 83–9

J

journal, keeping a 14, 29, 48, 53, 103

L

light, importance of 51, 57, 58
listening 39–43
Living Wills 91
logbook, keeping a 29

M

massage 21, 53, 101
meal preparation 58, 74, 98
mealtimes 74–8
meaningful activities 36–8, 39
medical treatment 44–9, 79–82
medications 12, 14, 18, 44, 46, 51, 60, 79–82, 96
    side effects 79, 81–2, 84
memory loss 11, 25, 27, 29, 30, 34, 42, 43
mirrors 72, 95
music 28, 34, 37, 53, 59, 61, 67, 76, 89, 101

O

oral hygiene 69–70

P

palliative care 102
paranoia 30, 60–2
personal care 65–73
Personal Care Book 23, 46, 67
personal documents 20
personal history 14, 45
planning 16, 17, 18, 28, 90–4, 100

privacy 67, 68, 71
pets 38, 61
physician, role of 14, 15, 16, 18, 27, 29, 44, 45, 46, 48, 51, 55, 59, 61, 63, 72, 78, 81, 82, 87, 88, 102
Power of Attorney 20, 91–4

R

reading 29, 30, 34, 59, 101, 103
record-keeping 11, 14, 29, 48, 53, 72, 79, 81, 82
Reminyl 80
research 28
resource materials 17, 20, 21, 23, 27, 46, 56, 62, 67, 96, 100, 101
respite for caregivers 18–23, 47–8, 59, 60, 69, 101
restlessness 30, 57–8, 75
reversal of symptoms 15, 16
routines, importance of 51, 52, 61, 65, 69, 70, 72, 74, 81, 99

S

Safely Home—Alzheimer Wandering Registry 21, 62, 96
safety 60, 62, 63, 69, 77, 95–9
self-esteem 10, 32, 37, 65
sexuality 83–9
sleep 59–60, 99
spirituality 32–5
stress for caregivers 10, 17, 20, 22, 52
sundowning. *See* restlessness
support groups 17, 19

T

television 40, 52, 57
Therapeutic Caregiving 56
touch, importance of 40, 41, 47, 53, 54, 76, 86, 101
travelling 55–6
trust, establishment of a 93–4
tube-feeding 78

V

visiting 21, 39, 46–8

W

wandering 21, 45, 59, 62–4
washroom, using 50, 59, 62, 63, 72–3, 97–8
Ways to Help 20
Wills 20, 71

The Author

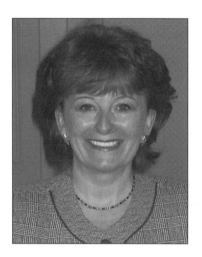

Judith McCann-Beranger, B.A., B.Ed., M.A., CCFE, has been involved in working with and on behalf of families for all of her adult life. She is an educator, counsellor, and mediator who has been recognized for her work provincially and nationally. Judy is the President of Family Mediation Canada, and is a Past President of Family Service Canada. Judy is currently the Executive Director of the Alzheimer Society of Prince Edward Island and has donated all the proceeds of this best seller book, over $100,000 to date, to this Society. She and her husband Greg live in Charlottetown.